Therapeutic and Advanced ERCP

Guest Editor

MICHEL KAHALEH, MD

GASTROINTESTINAL ENDOSCOPY CLINICS OF NORTH AMERICA

www.giendo.theclinics.com

Consulting Editor
CHARLES J. LIGHTDALE, MD

July 2012 • Volume 22 • Number 3

SAUNDERS an imprint of ELSEVIER, Inc.

W.B. SAUNDERS COMPANY
A Division of Elsevier Inc.

1600 John F. Kennedy Blvd. ● Suite 1800 ● Philadelphia, Pennsylvania 19103-2899

http://www.giendo.theclinics.com

GASTROINTESTINAL ENDOSCOPY CLINICS OF NORTH AMERICA Volume 22, Number 3
July 2012 ISSN 1052-5157, ISBN-13: 978-1-4557-4914-0

Editor: Kerry Holland
Developmental Editor: Donald Mumford

Gastrointestinal Endoscopy Clinics of North America (ISSN 1052-5157) is published quarterly by Elsevier Inc., 360 Park Avenue South, New York, NY 10010-1710. Months of issue are January, April, July, and October. Business and Editorial Offices: 1600 John F. Kennedy Blvd., Suite 1800, Philadelphia, PA, 19103-2899. Periodicals postage paid at New York, NY and additional mailing offices. Subscription prices are $315.00 per year for US individuals, $441.00 per year for US institutions, $168.00 per year for US students and residents, $351.00 per year for Canadian individuals, $538.00 per year for Canadian institutions, $445.00 per year for international individuals, $538.00 per year for international institutions, and $234.00 per year for Canadian and foreign students/residents. To receive student/resident rate, orders must be accompanied by name of affiliated institution, date of term, and the *signature* of program/residency coordinator on institution letterhead. Orders will be billed at individual rate until proof of status is received. Foreign air speed delivery is included in all *Clinics* subscription prices. All prices are subject to change without notice. **POSTMASTER:** Send address change to *Gastrointestinal Endoscopy Clinics of North America*, Elsevier Health Sciences Division, Subscription Customer Service, 3251 Riverport Lane, Maryland Heights, MO 63043. **Customer Service: 1-800-654-2452 (US). From outside the United States, call 1-314-447-8871. Fax: 1-314-447-8029. E-mail: JournalsCustomerService-usa@elsevier.com (for print support) or JournalsOnlineSupport-usa@elsevier.com (for online support).**

Reprints. For copies of 100 or more, of articles in this publication, please contact the Commercial Reprints Department, Elsevier Inc., 360 Park Avenue South, New York, NY 10010-1710. Tel. (212) 633-3812; Fax: (212) 482-1935; E-mail: reprints@elsevier.com.

Gastrointestinal Endoscopy Clinics of North America is covered in *Excerpta Medica, MEDLINE/PubMed (Index Medicus), and MEDLINE/MEDLARS.*

Printed and bound by CPI Group (UK) Ltd, Croydon, CR0 4YY
Transferred to Digital Print 2012

Contributors

CONSULTING EDITOR

CHARLES J. LIGHTDALE, MD
Professor, Department of Medicine, Columbia University Medical Center, New York, New York

GUEST EDITOR

MICHEL KAHALEH, MD, AGAF, FACG, FASGE
Professor of Clinical Medicine, Chief, Endoscopy, Medical Director Pancreas Program, Division of Gastroenterology and Hepatology, Department of Medicine, Weill Cornell Medical College, New York, New York

AUTHORS

JOHN BAILLIE, MB, ChB, FRCP, FASGE
Consulting Gastroenterologist, Carteret Medical Group, Morehead City, North Carolina

ROBERT L. BARCLAY, MD, MSc, FRCP
Assistant Professor of Clinical Medicine, University of Illinois College of Medicine; Rockford Gastroenterology Associates, Rockford, Illinois

CALVIN H.Y. CHAN, MBBS, FRACP
Division of Gastroenterology, St Paul's Hospital, The University of British Columbia, Vancouver, Canada

PETER B. COTTON, MD, FRCS, FRCP
Professor of Medicine, Department of Digestive Disease Center, Medical University of South Carolina, Charleston, South Carolina

PETER V. DRAGANOV, MD
Professor of Medicine, Section of Hepatobiliary Diseases, Division of Gastroenterology, Hepatology and Nutrition, Department of Medicine, University of Florida, Gainesville, Florida

JEAN-MARC DUMONCEAU, MD, PhD
Division of Gastroenterology and Hepatology, Geneva University Hospitals, Geneva, Switzerland

MARTIN L. FREEMAN, MD, FACG, FASGE
Professor of Medicine, Interim Director, Gastroenterology, Hepatology and Nutrition; Director Pancreaticobiliary Endoscopy Fellowship, University of Minnesota, Minneapolis, Minnesota

JAQUELINA M. GOBELET, MD
Gastroenterologist and Endoscopist Staff, The Latin American Advanced Gastrointestinal Endoscopy Training Center, Endoscopy Division, Clínica Alemana Santiago; Professor at the Universidad del Desarrollo, Santiago de Chile, Chile

TSUYOSHI HAMADA, MD
Department of Gastroenterology, Graduate School of Medicine, The University of Tokyo, Tokyo, Japan

KENJI HIRANO, MD, PhD
Department of Gastroenterology, Graduate School of Medicine, The University of Tokyo, Tokyo, Japan

HIROYUKI ISAYAMA, MD, PhD
Assistant Professor, Department of Gastroenterology, Graduate School of Medicine, The University of Tokyo, Tokyo, Japan

MICHEL KAHALEH, MD, AGAF, FACG, FASGE
Professor of Clinical Medicine, Chief, Endoscopy, Medical Director Pancreas Program, Division of Gastroenterology and Hepatology, Department of Medicine, Weill Cornell Medical College, New York, New York

KAZUMICHI KAWAKUBO, MD, PhD
Department of Gastroenterology, Graduate School of Medicine, The University of Tokyo, Tokyo, Japan

HIROFUMI KOGURE, MD, PhD
Department of Gastroenterology, Graduate School of Medicine, The University of Tokyo, Tokyo, Japan

KAZUHIKO KOIKE, MD, PhD
Department of Gastroenterology, Graduate School of Medicine, The University of Tokyo, Tokyo, Japan

YOUSUKE NAKAI, MD, PhD
Department of Gastroenterology, Graduate School of Medicine, The University of Tokyo, Tokyo, Japan

CLAUDIO NAVARRETE, MD
Chairman and Professor, The Latin American Advanced Gastrointestinal Endoscopy Training Center, Endoscopy Division, Clínica Alemana Santiag; Professor at the Universidad del Desarrollo, Santiago de Chile, Chile

DAVINDERBIR S. PANNU, MD
Division of Internal Medicine, Department of Medicine, Internal Medicine Residency Program, University of Florida, Gainesville, Florida

SANDEEP N. PATEL, DO
Associate Professor of Medicine and Pediatrics, Department of Medicine, University of Texas Health Science Center at San Antonio, San Antonio, Texas

MANUEL PEREZ-MIRANDA, MD
Associate Professor of Medicine, Division of Gastroenterology and Hepatology, Hospital Universitario Rio Hortega, Valladolid University Medical School, Valladolid, Spain

LAURA ROSENKRANZ, MD
Assistant Professor of Medicine, Department of Medicine, University of Texas Health Science Center at San Antonio, San Antonio, Texas

NAOKI SASAHIRA, MD, PhD
Department of Gastroenterology, Graduate School of Medicine, The University of Tokyo, Tokyo, Japan

AMRITA SETHI, MD
Assistant Professor of Clinical Medicine, Division of Gastroenterology and Hepatology, Interventional Endoscopy, Columbia University College of Physicians and Surgeons, New York, New York

INDU SRINIVASAN, MD
PGY 2 Internal Medicine Resident, Department of Internal Medicine, Saint Vincent Hospital, Worcester, Massachusetts

JENNIFER J. TELFORD, MD, MPH, FRCPC
Clinical Associate Professor of Medicine, Division of Gastroenterology, St Paul's Hospital, The University of British Columbia, Vancouver, Canada

OSAMU TOGAWA, MD, PhD
Department of Gastroenterology, Saitama Medical University International Medical Center, Saitama, Japan

TAKESHI TSUJINO, MD, PhD
Department of Gastroenterology, Graduate School of Medicine, The University of Tokyo, Tokyo, Japan

Contents

Over the last 40 years, endoscopic retrograde cholangiopancreatography
(ERCP) has evolved from being a purely diagnostic to a primarily therapeutic procedure. The 2 recent developments in ERCP-based stricture management include the increased use of cholangioscopy-guided sampling
and self-expandable metal stents. The role of ERCP in pancreatic diseases
continues to evolve; ERCP-based pancreatic therapy requires advanced
endoscopic expertise and is associated with a high rate of postprocedure
complications. Therefore, a multidisciplinary team approach at a center
with expertise in pancreatic therapy should serve as a basis for very careful
patient selection.

For most ERCP endoscopists, the greatest hurdle to a successful procedure is deep cannulation of the bile duct. This article explores basic cannulation technique, then reviews a variety of instruments and techniques
designed to increase the average endoscopist's success rate. Expert
ERCP endoscopists have a few favorite techniques that have proved reliable over time. The most frequently used ones are highlighted in this review.

Stones in biliary and pancreatic ducts are entities that plague hundreds of
thousands of patients worldwide every year. Symptoms can be mild (pain)
to life threatening (cholangitis, severe acute pancreatitis). In the last few
decades, management of these stones has transitioned from exclusively
surgical to now predominantly endoscopic techniques. This article reviews
the evolution of endoscopic techniques used in the management of stones
in the common bile duct and pancreatic duct.

Developments in endoscopic retrograde cholangioscopy provide multiple
new advanced methods of biliary imaging. Cholangioscopy provides

direct visualization of epithelium with white light as well as advanced modalities, such as narrow band imaging and autofluorescence. In vivo histologic images can be achieved with confocal endomicroscopy. Cross-sectional imaging is also possible with intraductal ultrasonography and optical coherence tomography. This article describes these advanced imaging techniques, which can be used together to assist in the diagnosis of biliary strictures and lesions.

Sampling at ERCP may be performed at the level of the papilla or of the biliopancreatic ducts. Samples collected at the level of the biliopancreatic ducts allow for diagnosing malignancy with a specificity close to 100% but present a moderate sensitivity in most studies. In this article, the different aspects of sampling at ERCP are discussed, and a special focus is placed on the means that are routinely available to the endoscopist for obtaining a high sensitivity for the diagnosis of malignancy.

Endoscopic biliary stent placement is widely accepted as palliation for malignant biliary obstruction or as a treatment of benign biliary stricture. Although various biliary stent designs have become available since self-expandable metallic stents were introduced, no single ideal stent has been developed. An ideal stent should be patent until death, or surgery, in patients with resectable malignant biliary obstruction. Fewer complications, maneuverability, cost-effectiveness, and removability are also important factors. Alternatively, should we develop a novel method for biliary drainage other than biliary stenting via endoscopic retrograde cholangiopancreatography? This article reviews the current status of biliary stenting for malignant biliary obstructions.

Endoscopic retrograde cholangiopancreatography (ERCP) is the standard approach to gaining access to the biliary and pancreatic ductal systems. However, in a small subset of cases anatomic constraints imposed by disease states or abnormal anatomy preclude ductal access via conventional ERCP. With the advent of endoscopic ultrasonography (EUS), with its unique capabilities of accurate imaging and ductal access via transmural puncture, there is now an alternative to surgical and percutaneous radiologic approaches in situations inaccessible to ERCP: endosonographic cholangiopancreatography (ESCP). This article reviews the background, technical details, published experience, and role of ESCP in clinical practice.

Endoscopic retrograde cholangiopancreatography (ERCP) is the first-line management in most situations when a benign biliary stricture is suspected. Although management principles are similar in all subgroups, the anticipated response rates, need for ancillary medical and endoscopic approaches, and use of less proven strategies vary between differing causes. Exclusion of malignancy should always be a focus of management. Newer endoscopic techniques such as endoscopic ultrasound, cholangioscopy, confocal endomicroscopy, and metal biliary stenting are increasingly complementing traditional ERCP techniques in achieving long-term sustained stricture resolution. Surgery remains a definitive management alternative when a prolonged trial of endoscopic therapy does not achieve treatment goals.

Video of a plastic biliary stent exchange in a patient with a benign distal biliary stricture secondary to chronic pancreatitis accompanies this article.

The treatment of common biliary duct injuries after surgery is a permanent challenge for physicians, and management by a multidisciplinary team is often required. The endoscopic approach is a valuable tool because it is able to assess the problem and also provide a therapeutic option for both fistulas and stenosis of the biliary tree. This article discusses the endoscopic management of postsurgical injuries of the common bile duct and discusses the application of practical tools.

Strictures at the hilum are caused by varied conditions and don't usually become symptomatic until obstructing the bile ducts, thus posing diagnostic and therapeutic challenges to physicians. ERCP is the method of choice for tissue diagnosis and decompression. MRCP or MRI with dedicated liver protocol provides a unique ability to visualize anatomy and promote procedure planning. In patients with unresectable tumor, endoscopic biliary stenting is a palliative approach. Percutaneous or EUS-guided approach is reserved for endoscopic failure. Various new modalities such as radiotherapy, chemotherapy and Photodynamic therapy have emerged but their superiority needs to be confirmed with Randomized Control studies.

Endoscopic retrograde cholangiopancreatography (ERCP) is now almost exclusively a therapeutic modality for pancreatic as well as biliary disorders. ERCP alone or with associated pancreatic and biliary therapy can cause a spectrum of mild and severe complications, including pancreatitis, hemorrhage, perforation, and cardiopulmonary events. Understanding of complications of ERCP has progressed substantially in the past decade, including widespread adoption of standardized consensus-based definitions of complications, large multicenter multivariate studies that have permitted clearer understanding of patient and technique-related risk factors for complications, and introduction of new technical approaches to minimize risks of ERCP.

Endoscopic retrograde cholangiopancreatography (ERCP) has become enormously popular throughout the world because of its proven value in the management of patients with known and suspected biliary and pancreatic disease. The results of ERCP are operator dependent, and there are significant risks. Adverse events are more likely when procedures are performed by endoscopists with inadequate training and experience. The best outcomes should occur when procedures are done for the best reasons, using optimal techniques in an ideal environment and a well-trained team, conscious of the risks and the ways to minimize them. This article discusses these intertwining elements of ERCP.

GASTROINTESTINAL ENDOSCOPY CLINICS OF NORTH AMERICA

RELATED INTEREST

Clinics in Liver Disease, May 2012 (Vol. 16, No. 2)
Approach to Consultations for Patients with Liver Disease
Steven L. Flamm, MD, *Guest Editor*

Foreword
Therapeutic and Advanced ERCP
Is Rapidly Progressing

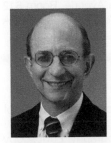

Charles J. Lightdale, MD
Consulting Editor

From the first published report of endoscopic cannulation of the ampulla of Vater by W.S. McCune and colleagues[1] in 1968, and the remarkable demonstrations of Oi and colleagues[2] using improved duodenoscopes in 1970, endoscopic retrograde cholangiopancreatography (ERCP) has made amazing progress. As radiological imaging (primarily computed tomography and magnetic resonance imaging) advanced in parallel, and special endoscopic ancillary tools for ERCP were developed, the focus has shifted strongly from mainly diagnostic to therapeutic uses for ERCP. During ERCP, the combined utilization of endoscopy and fluoroscopy to access and operate within the ductal systems of the liver and the pancreas has proven to be extremely powerful. Arguably, the most difficult and yet the most exciting of all procedures in gastrointestinal endoscopy today, therapeutic ERCP, has assumed a major role in managing diseases of the biliary tree and the pancreas.

I am particularly grateful that Michel Kahaleh, an internationally recognized authority in ERCP, is the guest editor for this issue of the *Gastrointestinal Endoscopy Clinics of North America* on the subject of "Therapeutic and Advanced Endoscopic Retrograde Cholangiopancreatography." Dr Kahaleh brings his knowledge, skills, experience, and energy to this topic and has enlisted an extraordinary group of fellow experts to participate. Everyone who performs ERCP, wrapped in lead from neck to knees, probing the ampulla of Vater through an endoscope while looking at both endoscopic and

Gastrointest Endoscopy Clin N Am 22 (2012) xiii–xiv
doi:10.1016/j.giec.2012.05.011
giendo.theclinics.com
1052-5157/12/$ – see front matter © 2012 Elsevier Inc. All rights reserved.

fluoroscopic screens, should read this issue, which highlights the present and rapidly developing future of this fascinating procedure.

Charles J. Lightdale, MD
Department of Medicine
Columbia University Medical Center
161 Fort Washington Avenue, Room 812
New York, NY 10032, USA

E-mail address:
CJL18@columbia.edu

REFERENCES

1. McCune WS, Shorb PE, Moscovitz H. Endoscopic cannulation of the ampulla of Vater: a preliminary report. Ann Surg 1968;167:752–6.
2. Oi I, Kobayashi S, Kondo T. Endoscopic pancreatocholangiography. Endoscopy 1970;2:103.

Preface

Therapeutic and Advanced Endoscopic Retrograde Cholangiopancreatography

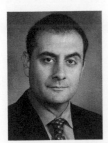

Michel Kahaleh, MD, AGAF
Guest Editor

Endoscopic retrograde cholangiopancreatography (ERCP) has seen dramatic changes within the last two decades. It went from being a diagnostic technique to a unique therapeutic and imaging platform. Alongside the expending indications of ERCP, major progress in instrumentations, devices, and tools has been made. New concepts have been generated regarding treating but most importantly preventing complications of ERCP, while advanced imaging technologies have taken the diagnostic possibilities to another level. The addition of novel stents, ablation therapy, and endoscopic ultrasound-guided ERCP has completely changed the field for years to come, while the medico-legal implications have added a whole new dimension by emphasizing indications and expertise.

This edition of *Gastrointestinal Endoscopy Clinics of North America* gathers outstanding material from expert opinions and articles focused on therapeutic and advanced ERCP. We truly hope you find this edition unique in offering the most appropriate and cutting-edge options to your patients.

Michel Kahaleh, MD, AGAF
Division of Gastroenterology and Hepatology
Department of Medicine
Weill Cornell Medical College
1305 York Avenue, 4th Floor
New York, NY 10021, USA

E-mail address:
mkahaleh@gmail.com

Gastrointest Endoscopy Clin N Am 22 (2012) xv
doi:10.1016/j.giec.2012.06.001
1052-5157/12/$ – see front matter © 2012 Elsevier Inc. All rights reserved.

giendo.theclinics.com

Therapeutic Endoscopic Retrograde Cholangiopancreatography and Instrumentation

Davinderbir S. Pannu, MD[a], Peter V. Draganov, MD[b],*

KEYWORDS

- Endoscopic retrograde cholangiopancreatography • ERCP • ERCP devices
- Short-wire ERCP devices

KEY POINTS

- Endoscopic retrograde cholangiopancreatography (ERCP) has become mainly a therapeutic procedure.
- The indications for therapeutic ERCP have significantly expanded.
- Short-wire ERCP device platforms have gained acceptance in everyday practice.
- The main perceived benefit from the use of short-wire instrumentation is the ability of the endoscopist to control the guide wire.
- The main benefit of the long-wire platform is its enormous flexibility given the larger number of devices available.
- A limited number of trials have directly compared the performance characteristics of short versus long-wire systems. Therefore the ultimate decision for the use of a specific device should be tailored to the case specifics, the endoscopist's expertise, and the availability of the trained assistant.

INTRODUCTION

Endoscopic retrograde cholangiopancreatography (ERCP) was introduced more than 40 years ago[1] as a purely diagnostic procedure, but over the years has evolved as the primary therapeutic tool for the management of pancreatic and

Disclosure: D.S. Pannu has no relationship with any company that has financial interest in this subject; P.V. Draganov is consultant for Boston Scientific Corporation and Cook Medical.
[a] Division of Internal Medicine, Department of Medicine, Internal Medicine Residency program, University of Florida, 1600 SW Archer Road, Gainesville, FL 32610-0214, USA; [b] Section of Hepatobiliary Diseases, Division of Gastroenterology, Hepatology and Nutrition, Department of Medicine, University of Florida, Box 100214, Room HD-602, Gainesville, FL 32610-0214, USA
* Corresponding author.
E-mail address: Peter.Draganov@medicine.ufl.edu

Gastrointest Endoscopy Clin N Am 22 (2012) 401–416
doi:10.1016/j.giec.2012.05.003
1052-5157/12/$ – see front matter © 2012 Elsevier Inc. All rights reserved.

biliary ductal disorders.[2,3] This article presents a comprehensive review of the current therapeutic ERCP indications and interventions, and recent advances in ERCP instrumentation.

BILIARY TRACT DISEASES

The indications for therapeutic ERCP for biliary tract disorders are summarized in **Box 1**. The 2 main indications are therapy for choledocholithiasis and biliary strictures.[3,4]

Choledocholithiasis

Indications for ERCP
Patients with suspected choledocholithiasis can be stratified as having low, intermediate, or high probability for common bile duct (CBD) stones based on clinical criteria

---

Box 1
Indications for therapeutic ERCP

Biliary

Choledocholithiasis

- High preoperative probability
- Definitive diagnosis before surgery
- Intraoperatively diagnosed bile duct stones

Postoperative biliary leaks

Biliary strictures

- Benign
- Malignant

Pancreatic

Chronic pancreatitis

- Strictures
- Stones

Pancreatic pseudocyst

Peripancreatic fluid collections

- In patient with prior history of pancreatitis

Acute pancreatitis

- Acute biliary pancreatitis
- Recurrent acute pancreatitis

Pancreatic ductal strictures

- Benign
- Malignant

Sphincter of Oddi dysfunction

- Type I
- Type II

Ampullary adenoma

(bilirubin elevation, dilation of the CBD, presence of cholangitis).[5,6] Patients with gall-bladder in situ and low probability for CBD stones should directly undergo laparoscopic cholecystectomy with consideration for intraoperative cholangiogram (IOC). Patients in the intermediate probability group should undergo preoperative evaluation with endoscopic ultrasonography (EUS) or magnetic resonance cholangiopancreatography (MRCP). Finally, patients in the high-probability group should undergo preoperative ERCP.

ERCP is the primary tool for treatment of documented choledocholithiasis if the stones are detected before or after laparoscopic cholecystectomy.[6,7] Some controversy exists on the possible management strategies of bile duct stones detected at the time of laparoscopic cholecystectomy. Systematic review of randomized controlled studies showed that there was no significant difference between laparoscopic and ERCP clearance of CBD stones.[8] Nevertheless, postoperative ERCP is the preferred method for treatment of CBD stones detected on IOC in the United States, because of its wide availability on the backdrop of relatively sparse surgical expertise in laparoscopic CBD exploration.

Instrumentation
Approximately 90% to 95% of CBD stones can usually be removed after endoscopic sphincterotomy by using balloon-tipped catheters or standard baskets. Larger stones are that difficult to remove may require specialized devices and techniques. If the main problem is that the stone is difficult to capture in the basket then a wire-guided, rotating, or multiwire basket can be applied.[9] For large stones, mechanical lithotripsy with a basket-type device has been traditionally used.[9] More recently the technique of using large (>12 mm) balloon dilation of the ampullary orifice after biliary sphincterotomy has gained popularity because of its simplicity, immediate availability, and high success rate.[7,10] Of note, no increase in incidence of post-ERCP pancreatitis was observed.[7,10] Although cholangioscopy-based lithotripsy with electrohydraulic lithotripsy (EHL) or laser has been available for more than 30 years, it just recently became feasible to use on a routine basis in everyday practice with the introduction of the SpyGlass Direct Visualization System (Boston Scientific Corporation, Natick, MA, USA) (**Fig. 1**).[11,12] SpyGlass-guided lithotripsy for bile duct stones that are difficult to remove has been shown to provide a high rate of stone clearance and low incidence of complications.[11,12] The cumbersome technique of mechanical lithotripsy can be avoided in most cases.[11]

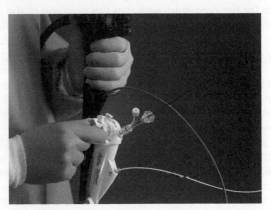

Fig. 1. Boston Scientific SpyGlass cholangioscope attached to the standard duodenoscope. (*Courtesy of* Boston Scientific Corporation, Marlborough, MA; with permission.)

Biliary Strictures

Indications for ERCP

ERCP is routinely done for evaluation of both benign and malignant biliary strictures because it can establish definitive tissue diagnosis and at the same time provide biliary drainage.[5,13] The most common causes of benign biliary strictures are postoperative defect, chronic pancreatitis, trauma, and cholangiopathy (eg, primary or secondary sclerosing cholangitis). Malignant strictures are most frequently due to pancreatic cancer, ampullary cancer, cholangiocarcinoma, gallbladder cancer, and metastatic malignant lymphadenopathy.

Instrumentation

Various ERCP-based sampling modalities are available to establish the specific etiology of the stricture.[14,15] More recently, the use of cholangioscopy-guided mini-forceps biopsy has been shown to increase the yield of ERCP-based sampling.[16]

A multitude of stents for ERCP-based biliary drainage is commercially available.[17] The choice of stent is determined by several factors including the etiology of the stricture, location of the lesion in the biliary tree (eg, distal versus proximal), patient prognosis, and the availability and cost of the specific device.

For benign biliary strictures, the standard endoscopic strategy for years has been to insert multiple plastic 10F stents over a period of 1 year with stent exchanges every 3 months.[18] This strategy is highly effective for postoperative strictures with results in the range of 70% to 80%,[19] but has been shown to have a relatively lower success rate for chronic pancreatitis–associated CBD stenosis (20%–30%). The main limitation of the treatment with multiple plastic stents is the need for multiple procedures over a long period of time and the relatively high incidence of cholangitis owing to stent occlusion.[20] More recently, the use of fully covered metal stents has shown promising short-term results for the treatment of benign biliary strictures.[21–26] The results of the long-term outcome studies that are currently under way are eagerly awaited.

Placement of a biliary stent in malignant obstruction is mostly palliative. For palliation purposes metal stents have been shown to be superior to plastic stents, because of their lower occlusion rate with the resulting lower incidence of cholangitis and need for stent exchanges.[20] Although no uniform consensus exists, in general partially covered or fully covered stents are preferred for distal biliary obstruction, whereas uncovered metal stents are used for proximal lesions. In the past, insertion of plastic stents was routinely done as a bridge to surgery in resectable patients with jaundice. The main rationale for the procedure was that the insertion of the stent would lead to resolution of the jaundice and provide for improvement in nutritional status of the patient, which may ultimately enhance surgical outcomes. Surprisingly a recent randomized study demonstrated worse outcomes in patients with pancreatic cancer who underwent preoperative ERCP biliary drainage with plastic stent compared with patients who went directly to surgery.[27] At present, one can consider sending patients directly to surgery without preoperative ERCP biliary drainage if the surgery can be done in a timely fashion (7–10 days from presentation) and the patient has a moderate degree of jaundice (total bilirubin <15 mg/dL).

Because bare and partially covered metal stents are very difficult and more frequently impossible to remove, until recently their deployment was reserved for patients with established tissue diagnosis of malignancy who were not considered to be surgical candidates. With the recent availability of fully covered metal stents, a new paradigm is emerging for the management of distal biliary strictures that appear to be malignant but without definitive tissue diagnosis available. The main premise is to insert a fully covered stent at the index ERCP. If the patient is later determined to have malignancy and is a surgical candidate, the stent can be easily removed at the time of surgery.[28] Alternatively, the patients who have malignant biliary obstruction and are not surgical candidates can be followed clinically with no further interventions because the majority will be effectively palliated with the fully covered metal stent. Finally, in patients with benign disease the metal stent can be removed endoscopically at a later date and the stricture reevaluated at that time. The viability of the described strategy has to be validated by further studies.

PANCREATIC DISEASES

Pancreatic diseases present an array of disorders that are very challenging to manage. The main indications for therapeutic ERCP for pancreatic disorders are summarized in **Box 1**. At present, ERCP is mostly used for the management of painful chronic pancreatitis (CP), pancreatic pseudocysts, peripancreatic fluid collections, and pancreatic duct disruption.[3,4] It seems prudent to observe the following guiding principles when considering endoscopic pancreatic therapy. (1) ERCP-based pancreatic therapy requires advanced endoscopic expertise and is associated with a high rate of postprocedure complications.[3,29] Therefore, one should maximize the use of noninvasive imaging before considering ERCP. (2) The availability of interventional EUS and extracorporeal shock-wave lithotripsy (ESWL) is highly desirable for achieving optimal outcomes. (3) A multidisciplinary team approach should serve as a basis for very careful patient selection.

Chronic Pancreatitis

Indications

ERCP can be used in establishing the diagnosis of CP, but currently its role is mostly in providing a platform for pancreatic ductal therapy in patients with painful CP.[30,31] The main goal of ERCP in the setting of CP is to overcome pancreatic duct obstruction caused by pancreatic duct strictures or stones. However, there have been no published validated guidelines for defining significant obstruction, or methodology for assessing patients before treatment and then judging the efficacy of that treatment. A multitude of retrospective and prospective case series on the role of ERCP-based therapy for CP has been published, but high-quality prospective randomized studies are lacking. The 2 randomized controlled trials published to date, comparing ERCP with surgery,[32,33] show superior results with the surgical approach, but both studies have been extensively criticized for their multiple methodological shortcomings. Most experts will apply the less invasive ERCP-based therapy first and reserve surgery for patients who have failed endoscopy. Because at present no clear high-quality evidence is available on the best management approach, one should consider referring patients to a center with expertise in the management of CP. A multidisciplinary team including a therapeutic endoscopist, a pancreatic surgeon, and a pain-management specialist should carefully incorporate patient specifics into a unified management strategy.

Instrumentation

Unfortunately the availability of dedicated specialized ERCP devices for pancreatic therapy is limited to plastic pancreatic stents. All other devices were originally designed for biliary work, but in the vast majority of cases these can be used successfully in the pancreatic duct. For pancreatic duct stones the addition of ESWL can significantly increase the success rate of ductal stone clearance.[34,35] However, a randomized controlled trial conducted by Dumonceau and colleagues[36] demonstrated that there was no difference between the patients with ESWL alone and patients treated with ESWL combined with ERCP. For treatment of pancreatic duct strictures, the traditional approach has been to dilate the stricture followed by placement of a single stent or multiple plastic stents for a prolonged period.[37] More recently, the placement of large plastic stents and fully covered biliary metal stents in the pancreatic duct has shown promising results.[38,39]

Pancreatic Duct Leaks

Although there are no comparative studies of surgical, medical, and endoscopic therapy for the treatment of pancreatic duct leaks, ERCP with pancreatic stenting has become the preferred approach to treat pancreatic duct disruption. Similar to biliary stenting, transpapillary pancreatic stents have been used with a high success rate for leaks attributable to acute or CP or postsurgical pancreatic duct fistulas.[40] ERCP-guided injection of N-butyl-2-cyanoacrylate to achieve closure of the pancreatic fistula has also been reported.[41]

Pancreatic Pseudocysts

Indications

Pancreatic pseudocyst can occur in the setting of acute pancreatitis or CP. Pseudocyst drainage is generally indicated for symptomatic pseudocyst, regardless of size.[42] ERCP can be used to perform transpapillary drainage; however, recently transluminal (transgastric or transduodenal) drainage has gained significant popularity. EUS-guided transmural drainage is considered an attractive option because of its ability to perform the cyst puncture under real-time EUS guidance and the ability to insert multiple large-bore plastic stents into the cyst cavity, thus providing a large tract for fluid evacuation. Not surprisingly, a randomized controlled study demonstrated that EUS-guided transluminal drainage was superior to the esophagogastroduodenoscopy-based technique.[43] To date, comparative studies of the technical success rates between transpapillary and transluminal drainage show conflicting results, and the choice is mostly dictated by endoscopists' preference.[44,45] A recently concluded prospective, randomized controlled trial by Park and colleagues[46] showed that the success rate of the initial technical procedure of EUS drainage was higher (94% vs 72%, $P = .039$) than that of the transpapillary approach. There was no significant difference in the long-term pseudocyst resolution between the two groups (89% vs 86%, $P = .696$). Although no randomized trials have compared endoscopic techniques with surgical ones, data from observational studies show a similar success rate with significantly decreased length of hospital stay in the endoscopy group.[47] A trend toward increasing use of endoscopic drainage and decreasing use of surgery has been well documented.[48]

Instrumentation

At present the devices used for ERCP-based transpapillary or EUS-based transluminal drainage are standard ERCP/EUS accessories. Despite the lack of special pseudocyst drainage accessories, the reported technical success has been very high, with rates greater than 90% reported by multiple series. Recently the first dedicated device for endoscopic pseudocyst drainage was introduced in the United States (NAVIX Access Device; Xlumena, Mountain View, CA, USA), with promising preliminary results.[49]

SHORT-WIRE AND LONG-WIRE ERCP DEVICE PLATFORMS

Arguably the most fundamental recent change in ERCP instrumentation has been the introduction of short-wire systems.[50,51] Guide wires are an indispensable part of ERCP and are used to gain and maintain access to the desired duct, and provide a platform for insertion or withdrawal of various devices. Long wires traditionally were exclusively used at the time of ERCP. The long length is dictated by the need to exchange various devices over the wire. The length of a typical long wire used for ERCP ranges from 420 to 480 cm. This excessive length creates several problems, including increased procedure and fluoroscopy time, because it may take longer to exchange various devices over the longer wire. Furthermore, because the assistant is in control of the wire and the physician is in control of the ERCP device, excellent communication between the physician and assistant is required. Failure to communicate and coordinate can lead to loss of access, more difficult cannulation, and problems with advancing the wire to a desired target. Moreover, it is not uncommon for the end of the long wire to touch the floor, leading to contamination. Finally, the assistant is challenged to perform multiple tasks at the same time, including advancing or retracting the wire, injecting dye, operating the device (inflating/deflating balloon, flexing/relaxing sphincterotome, and so forth), all while making sure that the end of the wire does not touch the floor.

To counter limitations that are associated with the use of the traditional long wires, the radically new concept of using the short wire was introduced. The main feature of all short-wire ERCP systems is the ability to lock the short wire in position to allow advancement or removal of various devices without displacement of the wire.[50,51] The perceived advantages of short-wire ERCP include reduced time for device exchange, stent insertion time, and need for wire adjustments (**Box 2**), all of which can further lead to decreased sedation requirements and decreased use of fluoroscopy. Furthermore, the locking mechanism secures the wire position, which can promote maintenance of ductal access, stricture access, and placement of multiple stents without recannulation. Of importance is that the short-wire platforms allow the endoscopist to be in control of the wire, which can lead to increased cannulation rate, decreased trauma to the ampulla, and decreased risk of post-ERCP pancreatitis. Finally, the ability of the endoscopist to control the wire makes the ultimate success of ERCP less dependent on the availability of a highly trained assistant.

At present, there are three available short-wire ERCP proprietary systems.[51] These systems integrate cannulation, sphincterotomy, balloon extraction, balloon dilation and biliary stenting devices. The key features of the three short wire platforms are summarized on **Table 1**.

The RX System, (Boston Scientific Corporation, Natick, MA, USA) was the first short-wire system introduced in 1999. This system incorporates three components: (1) The RX Locking Device that has an external lock which may accommodate fixation of 1 or 2 wires. The locking device is strapped to the scope shaft next to the biopsy port cap with a silastic band; (2) RX compatible devices include both open "tear away" channel design used with sphincterotomes and catheters as well as short-track designs used with cytology catheters, stone extraction balloons, dilating balloons and stents; (3) The last component includes the 260 cm long 0.035 inch or 0.025 inch wide Jagwire with a coated firm shaft, flexible hydrophilic leading tip and 2 colored markings, which aid in detection of wire movement[51] (**Fig. 2**). The 0.025 inch and 0.035 inch diameter wire should be used with their respective devices which are not interchangeable.

The Fusion platform (Cook Endoscopy; Winston Salem, NC, USA) was introduced in 2004. As in the RX Biliary System, the Fusion System incorporates both short-track and tear-away capabilities. The external wire lock fits and is snapped on the biopsy port enabling the locking of 1 or 2 wires (**Fig. 3**). A key feature of this platform includes a side port that has been placed in close proximity to the distal tip of the catheter or

---

Box 2
Potential advantages and disadvantages of the short-wire platforms

Advantages

1. Reduced exchange times
2. Reduced stent insertion times
3. Maintenance of ductal access
4. Reduction of sedation and fluoroscopy time
5. Increased endoscopist control of cannulation
6. Locking of wire in position to increase stability
7. Decreased rates of post-ERCP pancreatitis
8. Decreased trauma when ampullary surface is manipulated
9. Reduced rates of wire adjustments
10. Aids in stricture access
11. Allows placement of multiple stents (Fusion system only)

Disadvantages

1. Hydraulic exchange technique not plausible with RX system
2. Decreased pushability with the open-channel design of the RX system
3. Inability to flush channel for hydrophilic wire use (RX system)
4. Inability to use smaller than 0.035-in or angled wires when channel is torn after first device exchange (unless device is preloaded) (RX system)
5. Deterioration of the device after multiple exchanges (RX, Fusion systems)
6. No easy method for insertion of pancreatic stents (all systems)
7. No reliable method of locking wire (V-system)
8. Looping of wire between the biopsy port and the external locking device (RX, Fusion systems)
9. Poor guide-wire visibility (V-system)
10. Air and bile leakage causing increased soiling of operators (RX, Fusion systems)
11. Wires may suspend freely in air after being locked, jeopardizing operators (all systems)
12. Loss of visibility caused by decreased distention of the duodenum (RX, Fusion systems)

---

stent delivery system and a closed tear-away channel running the length of the catheter (as opposed to the open tear-away channel of the RX). The availability of a side port near the device tip allows for a true intraductal exchange (**Fig. 4**). With the intraductal exchange, the wire can be disengaged from the device while both are still within the biliary or pancreatic ducts. The device then can be withdrawn while the wire remains in place. The Fusion Metro guidewire is 0.035 inches in diameter and 185 cm in length with similar features as the Jagwire.[51] Studies from Europe and the US have shown improved placement of multiple plastic stents into the bile duct, or pseudocyst cavity minimizing the number of guidewires used and shortening the procedure duration[52,53] The ability to move from the short-wire to a long-wire configuration at any point during the procedure is a unique feature to the Fusion platform. This system also provides compatibility with all other systems including all straight tip or angled tip hydrophilic wires such as the Glidewire (Boston Scientific Corporation, Natick, MA, USA) available

Table 1
Comparison of the 3 short-wire platforms

Characteristics	RX System	Fusion System	V-System
Type of endoscope	Standard	Standard	V-scope
Type of lock	External at the biopsy port	External at the biopsy port	Internal lock design
Type of device	Open-channel tear-away	Closed-channel breakthrough	Closed-lumen device
Short-track technology	Yes	Yes	No
Wire length (cm)	260	185	270
Can be used with standard guide wires	Yes	Yes	Yes
Can be used with 0.025″ or 0.018″ or angled wires	No	Yes	Yes
Can be used with hydrophilic Glidewire	No	Yes	Yes
Ability to flush with wire channel	No	Yes	Yes
Intraductal exchange ability	No	Yes	No
Insertion of multiple stents without the need to recannulate	No	Yes	No
Physician control of wire	Yes	Yes	Yes
Pushability of short-wire devices	++	+++	+++

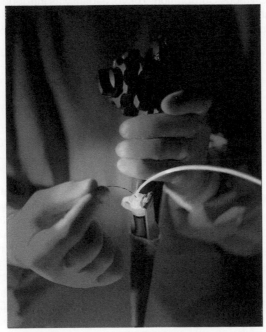

Fig. 2. Boston Scientific RX system with locking device positioned next to the biopsy channel cap and the wire separated from the shaft of the device through the "tear away" channel. (*Courtesy of* Boston Scientific Corporation, Marlborough, MA; with permission.)

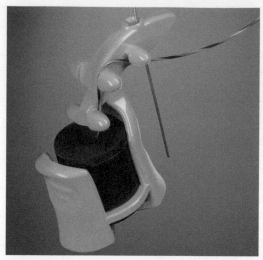

Fig. 3. Cook Medical Fusion platform wire lock fitting on the biopsy port cap with wire in locked position. (Permission for use granted by Cook Medical Incorporated, Bloomington, IN.)

commercially. Finally, the Fusion system provides dual platform capabilities and each device can be used exclusively in traditional long-wire or exclusively in short-wire configuration.

The V-System (Olympus Corporation, Tokyo, Japan) was introduced in 2005. This is the first modification of a duodenoscope for facilitation of wire exchanges. The elevator lever in this system includes a V-shaped groove and an increased angle of

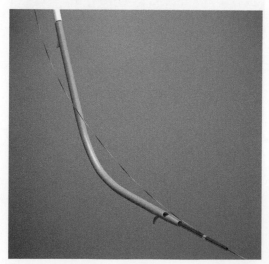

Fig. 4. Cook Medial Fusion platform stent delivery system with side port near the tip of the catheter allowing intraductal exchange and sequential deployment of multiple stents over the same wire. (Permission for use granted by Cook Medical Incorporated, Bloomington, IN.)

articulation in comparison to the standard Olympus TJF-160 series endoscopes (**Fig. 5**). This design promotes securing and locking of the short guidewire at the elevator level to reduce repositioning of the guidewire during accessory exchanges and importantly it obviates the need to affix an external lock at the scope biopsy port site. The groove described above acts as the internal wire lock allowing use of a catheter without a short-wire track. Therefore, the V-System devices are similar to the traditional long-wire devices at the leading end and the device shaft (closed channel lumen). The proximal (external) end of the V-System devices has a unique design called C-Hook.[51] The C-Hook allows the device handle to be attached to the proximal end of the duodenoscope (**Fig. 6**). This enables the endoscopist to maneuver the guidewire, inject contrast and manipulate the device handle while keeping a grip on the device control section. The main advantage of the C-Hook lies in that it is very easy for the endoscopist to relinquish control of the guidewire back to the assistant if needed. Recently a new generation of V-System duodenoscopes (TIF-180V) with better wire locking capabilities became commercially available in the US.

A recently concluded randomized controlled trial in the authors' institution compared the Fusion short-wire system and long-wire devices.[52] This study showed that the short-wire system provided for significantly faster mean device exchange time (125 vs 177 seconds; $P = .05$) and stent insertion time (135 vs 254 seconds; $P<.001$)

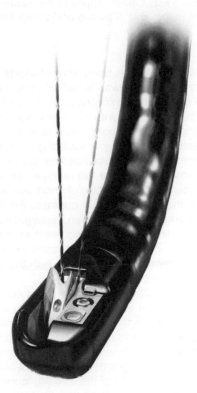

Fig. 5. Olympus V series side viewing duodenoscope with V shaped elevator allowing locking of the wire at the tip of the endoscope. (*Courtesy of* Olympus America, Inc., Center Valley, PA; with permission.)

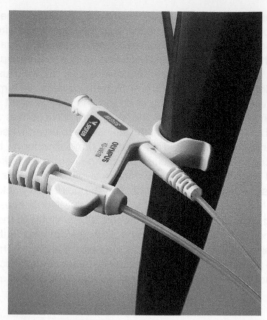

Fig. 6. Olympus sphincterotome with C-hook clipped to the handle of the endoscope allowing wire manipulation by the endoscopist. (*Courtesy of* Olympus America, Inc., Center Valley, PA; with permission.)

compared with the long-wire system. A trend toward shorter total procedure time, fluoroscopy time, and cannulation time was noted with the short-wire system, which however did not reach statistical significance. In an earlier study, Joyce and colleagues[53] compared the V-system with long-wire accessories, reporting very similar results to the findings of the authors' more recent study. Of note, although both studies demonstrated shorter device exchange times with the short-wire systems, they failed to demonstrate improved cannulation rate or decreased rate of post-ERCP pancreatitis, most likely due to the relatively small sample sizes. In the authors' opinion, the main benefit from the use of short-wire systems is the ability of the endoscopist to control the guide wire. By contrast, the main advantage of the long-wire platform is its enormous flexibility, given the larger number of devices available. Unfortunately, it will be very difficult to document improved patient outcomes (eg, increased cannulation rate, increased stricture access rate, decreased incidence of post-ERCP pancreatitis) comparing one platform with the other, because this will require a very large comparative trial.

Use of the short-wire platforms does not come without some limitations. Potential problems associated with short-wire use include decreased pushability owing to the open-channel design (RX), inability to flush the channel to facilitate use with a hydrophilic wire (RX), inability to use smaller than 0.035-in or angled wires after the channel is torn with the first device exchange (unless the device is preloaded) (RX), deterioration of the device after multiple exchanges (RX, Fusion), not being able to easily insert pancreatic stents (all), no reliable locking of the wire (V), looping of the wire between the biopsy port and the external locking device (RX, Fusion), and air and bile leakage that may lead to soiling of the operator and loss of visibility caused by decreased distention of the duodenum (RX and Fusion) (see **Box 2**). These disadvantages have kept the short-wire platforms from becoming universally accepted in everyday practice. Indeed, recently Coté and colleagues[54] conducted a national survey and showed that although a small majority of physicians prefer the short-wire platform (54%), a large minority still use the long wire (46%). Low-volume endoscopists (<50 ERCPs per year) favored the short-wire platform (59% vs 42%, $P = .003$) in a comparison with high-volume endoscopists (>200 ERCPs per year).

SUMMARY

ERCP is an important therapeutic tool for the management of pancreatobiliary diseases. ERCP is the procedure of choice for stone extraction in patients with choledocholithiasis and in patients with benign and malignant biliary strictures. The role of ERCP for the management of pancreatic diseases is increasing, but remains confined to major referral centers. Therapeutic ERCP is complex and technically demanding, and carries higher potential for serious complications in comparison with other endoscopic procedures. A multitude of ERCP devices is available, and thorough familiarity with their use is one of the crucial components of successful ERCP.

REFERENCES

1. Rabinov K, Simon M. Peroral cannulation of ampulla of Vater for direct cholangiography and pancreatography. Radiology 1965;85:693.
2. Parra-Membrives P, Díaz-Gómez D, Vilegas-Portero R, et al. Appropriate management of common bile duct stones: a RAND corporation/UCLA appropriateness method statistical analysis. Surg Endosc 2010;24(5):1187–94.
3. NIH state-of-the-science statement on endoscopic retrograde cholangiopancreatography (ERCP) for diagnosis and therapy. NIH Consens State Sci Statements 2002;19:1–26.
4. Adler DG, Baron TH, Davila RE, et al. ASGE guideline: the role of ERCP in diseases of the biliary tract and the pancreas. Gastrointest Endosc 2005;62(1):1.
5. Shiozawa S, Kim DH, Usui T, et al. Indication of endoscopic retrograde cholangiography by noninvasive predictive factors of common bile duct stones before laparoscopic cholecystectomy: a prospective clinical study. Surg Laparosc Endosc Percutan Tech 2011;21(1):28–32.
6. ASGE Standards of Practice Committee, Maple JT, Ben-Menachem T, et al. The role of endoscopy in the evaluation of suspected choledocholithiasis. Gastrointest Endosc 2010;71(1):1–9.
7. ASGE Standards of Practice Committee, Maple JT, Ikenberry SO, et al. The role of endoscopy in the management of choledocholithiasis. Gastrointest Endosc 2011;74(4):731–44 [Erratum appears in: Gastrointest Endosc 2012;75(1): 230–230, e14].
8. Martin DJ, Vernon DR, Toouli J. Surgical versus endoscopic treatment of bile duct stones. Cochrane Database Syst Rev 2006;2:CD003327.
9. DiSario J, Chuttani R, Croffie J, et al. Biliary and pancreatic lithotripsy devices. Gastrointest Endosc 2007;65(6):750–6.
10. Draganov PV, Evans W, Fazel A, et al. Large size balloon dilation of the ampulla after biliary sphincterotomy can facilitate endoscopic extraction of difficult bile duct stones. J Clin Gastroenterol 2009;43(8):782–6.
11. Draganov PV, Lin T, Chauhan S, et al. Prospective evaluation of the clinical utility of ERCP-guided cholangiopancreatoscopy with a new direct visualization system. Gastrointest Endosc 2011;73(5):971–9.

12. Chen YK, Parsi MA, Binmoeller KF, et al. Single-operator cholangioscopy in patients requiring evaluation of bile duct disease or therapy of biliary stones (with videos). Gastrointest Endosc 2011;74(4):805–14.
13. Moss AC, Morris E, Leyden J, et al. Malignant distal biliary obstruction: a systematic review and metaanalysis of endoscopic and surgical bypass results. Cancer Treat Rev 2007;33:213–21.
14. de Bellis M, Sherman S, Fogel EL, et al. Tissue sampling at ERCP in suspected malignant biliary strictures (part 1). Gastrointest Endosc 2002;56(4): 552–61.
15. de Bellis M, Sherman S, Fogel EL, et al. Tissue sampling at ERCP in suspected malignant biliary strictures (part 2). Gastrointest Endosc 2002;56(5):720–30.
16. Draganov PV, Chauhan S, Wagh MS, et al. Diagnostic accuracy of conventional and cholangioscopy-guided sampling of indeterminate biliary lesions at the time of ERCP: a prospective, long-term follow-up study. Gastrointest Endosc 2012; 75(2):347–53.
17. Somogyi L, Chuttani R, Croffie J, et al. Biliary and pancreatic stents. Gastrointest Endosc 2006;63(7):910–9.
18. Williams ED, Draganov PV. Endoscopic management of biliary strictures after liver transplantation. World J Gastroenterol 2009;15(30):3725–33.
19. Morelli J, Mulcahy HE, Willner IR, et al. Long-term outcomes for patients with post-liver transplant anastomotic biliary strictures treated by endoscopic stent placement. Gastrointest Endosc 2003;58(3):374–9.
20. Sejpal D. Advancements in biliary stenting. J Clin Gastroenterol 2012;46(3): 191–6.
21. Kahaleh M, Behm B, Clarke BW, et al. Temporary placement of covered self-expandable metal stents in benign biliary strictures: a new paradigm? Gastrointest Endosc 2008;67(3):446–54.
22. Poley JW, Cahen DL, Metselaar HJ, et al. A prospective group sequential study evaluating a new type of fully covered self-expandable metal stent for the treatment of benign biliary strictures (with video). Gastrointest Endosc 2012; 75(4):783–9.
23. van Boeckel PG, Vleggaar FP, Siersema PD. Plastic or metal stents for benign extrahepatic biliary strictures: a systematic review. BMC Gastroenterol 2009;9:96.
24. Srinivasan I, Kahaleh M. Biliary stents in the millennium. Adv Ther 2011;28(11): 960–72.
25. Bakhru MR, Kahaleh M. Expandable metal stents for benign biliary disease. Gastrointest Endosc Clin N Am 2011;21(3):447–62, viii.
26. Mahajan A, Ho H, Sauer B, et al. Temporary placement of fully covered self-expandable metal stents in benign biliary strictures: midterm evaluation (with video). Gastrointest Endosc 2009;70(2):303–9.
27. van der Gaag NA, Rauws EA, van Eijck CH, et al. Preoperative biliary drainage for cancer of the head of the pancreas. N Engl J Med 2010;362(2):129–37.
28. Siddiqui AA, Mehendiratta V, Loren D, et al. Fully covered self-expandable metal stents are effective and safe to treat distal malignant biliary strictures, irrespective of surgical resectability status. J Clin Gastroenterol 2011;45(9):824–7.
29. Freeman ML, DiSario JA, Nelson DB, et al. Risk factors for post-ERCP pancreatitis: a prospective, multicenter study. Gastrointest Endosc 2001;54(4): 425–34.
30. Calvo MM, Bujanda L, Calderón A, et al. Comparison between magnetic resonance cholangiopancreatography and ERCP for evaluation of the pancreatic duct. Am J Gastroenterol 2002;97:347–53.

31. Kowalczyk LM, Draganov PV. Endoscopic therapy for chronic pancreatitis: technical success, clinical outcomes, and complications. Curr Gastroenterol Rep 2009;11(2):111–8.
32. Dîte P, Ruzicka M, Zboril V, et al. A prospective, randomized trial comparing endoscopic and surgical therapy for chronic pancreatitis. Endoscopy 2003; 35(7):553–8.
33. Cahen DL, Gouma DJ, Nio Y, et al. Endoscopic versus surgical drainage of the pancreatic duct in chronic pancreatitis. N Engl J Med 2007;356(7):676–84.
34. Kozarek RA, Ball TJ, Patterson DJ, et al. Endoscopic pancreatic duct sphincterotomy: indications, technique, and analysis of results. Gastrointest Endosc 1994; 40:592–8.
35. Delhaye M, Vandermeeren A, Baize M, et al. Extracorporeal shock-wave lithotripsy of pancreatic calculi. Gastroenterology 1992;102:610–20.
36. Dumonceau JM, Costamagna G, Tringali A, et al. Treatment for painful calcified chronic pancreatitis: extracorporeal shock wave lithotripsy versus endoscopic treatment: a randomised controlled trial. Gut 2007;56(4):545–52.
37. Costamagna G, Bulajic M, Tringali A, et al. Multiple stenting of refractory pancreatic duct strictures in severe chronic pancreatitis: long-term results. Endoscopy 2006;38(3):254–9.
38. Sauer BG, Gurka MJ, Ellen K, et al. Effect of pancreatic duct stent diameter on hospitalization in chronic pancreatitis: does size matter? Pancreas 2009;38(7): 728–31.
39. Sauer B, Talreja J, Ellen K, et al. Temporary placement of a fully covered self-expandable metal stent in the pancreatic duct for management of symptomatic refractory chronic pancreatitis: preliminary data (with videos). Gastrointest Endosc 2008;68(6):1173–8.
40. Grobmyer SR, Hunt DL, Forsmark CE, et al. Pancreatic stent placement is associated with resolution of refractory grade C pancreatic fistula after left-sided pancreatectomy. Am Surg 2009;75(8):654–7 [discussion: 657–8].
41. Seewald S, Brand B, Groth S, et al. Endoscopic sealing of pancreatic fistula by using N-butyl-2-cyanoacrylate. Gastrointest Endosc 2004;59(4):463–70.
42. Habashi S, Draganov PV. Pancreatic pseudocyst. World J Gastroenterol 2009; 15(1):38–47.
43. Varadarajulu S, Christein JD, Tamhane A, et al. Prospective randomized trial comparing EUS and EGD for transmural drainage of pancreatic pseudocysts (with videos). Gastrointest Endosc 2008;68(6):1102–11.
44. Chahal P, Papachristou GI, Baron TH. Endoscopic transmural entry into pancreatic fluid collections using a dedicated aspiration needle without endoscopic ultrasound guidance: success and complication rates. Surg Endosc 2007;21:1726–32.
45. Varadarajulu S, Wilcox CM, Tamhane A, et al. Role of EUS in drainage of peripancreatic fluid collections not amenable for endoscopic transmural drainage. Gastrointest Endosc 2007;66:1107–19.
46. Park DH, lee SS, Moon SH, et al. Endoscopic ultrasound guided versus conventional transmural drainage for pancreatic pseudocyst: a prospective randomized trial. Endoscopy 2009;41(10):842–8.
47. Varadarajulu S, Lopes TL, Wilcox CM, et al. EUS versus surgical cystgastrostomy for management of pancreatic pseudocysts. Gastrointest Endosc 2008;68(4):649–55.
48. Varadarajulu S, Mel Wilcox C, Latif S, et al. Management of pancreatic fluid collections: a changing of the guard from surgery to endoscopy. Am Surg 2011;77(12):1650–5.

49. Itoi T, Binmoeller KF, Shah J, et al. Clinical evaluation of a novel lumen-apposing metal stent for endosonography-guided pancreatic pseudocyst and gallbladder drainage (with videos). Gastrointest Endosc 2012;75(4):870–6.
50. Reddy SC, Draganov PV. ERCP wire systems: the long and short of it. World J Gastroenterol 2009;15(1):55–60.
51. ASGE Technology Committee, Shah RJ, Somogyi L, et al. Short-wire ERCP systems [review]. Gastrointest Endosc 2007;66(4):650–7.
52. Draganov PV, Kowalczyk L, Fazel A, et al. Prospective randomized blinded comparison of a short-wire endoscopic retrograde cholangiopancreatography system with traditional long-wire devices. Dig Dis Sci 2010;55(2):510–5.
53. Joyce AM, Ahmad NA, Beilstein MC, et al. Multicenter comparative trial of the V-scope system for therapeutic ERCP. Endoscopy 2006;38(7):713–6.
54. Coté GA, Keswani RN, Jackson T, et al. Individual and practice differences among physicians who perform ERCP at varying frequency: a national survey. Gastrointest Endosc 2011;74(1):65–73, e12.

Advanced Cannulation Technique and Precut

John Baillie, MB, ChB

KEYWORDS

- Cannulation • ERCP • Papillotome • Needle knife papillotomy
- Biliary access techniques

KEY POINTS

- It probably takes 1000 ERCPs to become skilled at cannulation, and several thousand more to become an expert.
- The expert ERCP endoscopist must be able to innovate and adapt his or her technique to deal with unexpected and unfamiliar anatomy.
- ERCP has evolved into an almost entirely therapeutic modality, increasing the technical difficulty and requiring skill with guide wires, catheters, stents, and so forth.
- The "pull" papillotome has become the primary tool for ERCP cannulation.
- Needle knife papillotomy (NKP) should be taught to all serious students of ERCP, and no longer regarded as a high-risk procedure for experts only.
- The epidemic of obesity in the United States and the resulting explosion of bariatric (weight loss) surgery has created a population of patients whose bile ducts are endoscopically inaccessible using standard duodenoscopes and catheters.

INTRODUCTION

For most ERCP endoscopists, the greatest hurdle to a successful procedure is deep cannulation of the bile duct. It is like a potential energy "hump." What separates expert ERCP endoscopists from lesser ones is their ability to reliably cannulate the bile duct with the minimum of trauma to the duodenal papilla. There is a long learning curve involved, such is the variability in papillary and local gastrointestinal (GI) anatomy. This article explores basic cannulation technique, then reviews a variety of instruments and techniques designed to increase the average endoscopist's success rate (**Boxes 1** and **2**). Many of these techniques require access to the pancreatic duct (PD) for placement of a guide wire and stenting. Other techniques use precutting or needle knife papillotomy (NKP), "free hand," or down on to a guide wire or stent. It is the author's opinion that any sufficiency skilled and experienced ERCP endoscopist can overcome the great majority of local anatomic difficulties to obtain deep cannulation. There are many variables to consider when addressing success rates for biliary

Carteret Medical Group, 300 Penny Lane, Morehead City, NC 28557, USA
E-mail address: jbaillie@ccgh.org

Gastrointest Endoscopy Clin N Am 22 (2012) 417–434
doi:10.1016/j.giec.2012.05.010
1052-5157/12/$ – see front matter

giendo.theclinics.com

Box 1
Accessories for ERCP

Catheters
- Standard
- Tapered
- Steerable
- Cremer

Guide wires
- Coated and uncoated (nitinol, hybrid, hydrophilic)

Papillotomes
- Standard ("pull"-type)
- Needle knife
- Shark-fin
- Steerable
- Billroth-II

---

cannulation, including the training and experience of the operator, the technique used (eg, with or without precut papillotomy), local anatomic issues (eg, diverticula), familiarity with adjunctive techniques, such as cannulation over a stent or a guide wire, and so forth. The secret to being a skilled ERCP endoscopist is mastering a variety of techniques for deep access to the duct of choice. Prominent papillas, small papillas, upside-down papillas (in post-Billroth II gastrectomy afferent limbs), papillas inside diverticula, and those at the end of long Roux-en Y limbs all require a plan of attack and techniques tailored to the situation. The early ERCP experts could do a lot with a few tools, but their modern successors have many more accessories and techniques at their disposal. Professional golfers are permitted up to 14 clubs in their bags, but they tend to favor certain ones. Similarly, expert ERCP endoscopists have a few favorite techniques that have proved reliable over time. The most frequently used ones are highlighted in this review.

As Freeman and Guda[1] have pointed out, defining and measuring success at cannulation is problematic. How successful can a cannulation be considered if it is

---

Box 2
Adjunctive techniques for biliary and PD access

Placement of stent or guide wire in the PD to facilitate biliary cannulation

Precut papillotomy

NKP: "free-hand," fistulotomy, over-a-stent (or a guide wire)

Trans-septal (transpancreatic) sphincterotomy (Goff procedure)

Endoscopic scissors

Endoscopic dissection (cotton tip)

Papillectomy/ampullectomy

Needle tip (Cremer) catheter

Endoscopic ultrasound (EUS)-guided

---

followed by a serious, even life-threatening complication, such as perforation or necrotizing acute pancreatitis? Some clinical situations are recognized to carry a high risk of complications (eg, ERCP in suspected sphincter of Oddi dysfunction), whereas others are considered relatively safe (eg, bile duct stone removal in elderly patients with dilated ducts). The definition of success must take into account "intention to treat." Prior manipulation of the orifice, such as sphincterotomy, typically renders cannulation easier than instrumenting a virgin papilla. The perceived technical difficulty of ERCP is also a factor: Schutz and Abbott[2] proposed a 5-point scale of ERCP difficulty that has been useful to investigators looking at success and failure rates for this procedure. Perhaps the greatest value of such a scoring scale is that it makes novice endoscopists think twice before taking on challenging cases. In the past 20 years, ERCP has gone from being a largely diagnostic modality to an almost exclusively therapeutic one. The quality of modern abdominal imaging, by computed tomography (CT), magnetic resonance imaging (MRI), and endoscopic ultrasound (EUS) is such that a lot of the guesswork has gone out of investigating biliary and pancreatic disease. In modern ERCP practice, there should be few surprises for the endoscopist, who can and should use these high-resolution imaging techniques to map out the relevant anatomy and help plan the appropriate therapeutic intervention ahead of time. The risk of complications of ERCP, small as it may be in experienced hands, cannot be ignored in the interests of a "fishing trip." The comfort and safety of the patient must always be the top priority of the endoscopist.

STRAIGHT CATHETERS VERSUS PAPILLOTOMES

In the early days of ERCP, endoscopists started the procedure with a straight catheter. Indeed, I used to require that my trainees become adept at cannulation with a straight catheter before advancing to a papillotome, which is now most ERCP endoscopists' preferred first catheter.[3] Deep cannulation of the bile duct with a straight catheter requires accurate positioning from below the papilla to achieve the necessary axis; this is still a useful skill to attain. The fiscal reality of modern ERCP reimbursement no longer allows us the "luxury" of using multiple catheters, however: we now choose the one most likely to succeed. Some of the straight ERCP catheters are thin (tapered) and potentially traumatic to the papilla and ducts. I rarely use a straight catheter for biliary access. Papillotomes have the significant advantage of offering a variable angle for cannulation and subsequent manipulation to achieve deep access to the bile duct. Papillotomes have been developed that are "steerable," allowing the tip to be rotated in an arc.[4] Some endoscopists find these helpful, although experienced endoscopists have other ways to alter the tip direction without a steering mechanism. "Grooming" the papillotome tip, usually by twisting it counterclockwise, is a time-honored method of improving the cannulation axis, but this permanently deforms the catheter, which can prove problematic later in the procedure.

STANDARD CANNULATION TECHNIQUE

As a trainee, it is embarrassing to spend a long time struggling to cannulate, then have your teacher achieve deep cannulation on his or her first attempt. How do experts make this look easy? In ERCP, as with most hand-eye coordination skills, there is no substitute for experience. It probably takes at least 1000 cannulations to become truly comfortable with the technique, and several thousand more to become expert. Not every endoscopist has the spatial orientation and hand-eye coordination to reach this level. Most experienced ERCP teachers have come across trainees who fail to acquire the necessary skills even after many procedures. These novices are understandably frustrated with their lack of progress, and often blame their teachers for it. But without a "feel" for the 3-dimensional environment in which the ERCP endoscopist has to work, the attainment of expertise is unlikely. These individuals are rarely willing to acknowledge that ERCP is not for them, and continue to perform these procedures, often in the community where their annual volume of cases is low. This is a significant problem in the United States, where small numbers of cases done in training are often accepted for ERCP-credentialing purposes, and there is rarely a requirement to show maintenance of skills on periodic basis thereafter.

Every trainee who comes out of a gastroenterology fellowship intending to perform ERCP without further mentoring should be adept at selective cannulation. The growing recognition over the past decade that prophylactic stenting of the PD greatly reduces the risk of severe post-ERCP pancreatitis[5] makes the ability to reliably cannulate the duct of choice mandatory. The task of cannulation requires an organized approach. First, do not be in a hurry: take a good look at the main duodenal papilla and decide what the bile duct and PD axes are likely to be. This requires an unobstructed view, and control of duodenal motility by pharmacologic means if necessary. Are there any clues, like a biliary orifice gaping open, or a little trickle of bile, to guide your way? Has there been prior manipulation of the papilla (eg, endoscopic sphincterotomy) that will make cannulation easy, or easier? If the patient has had a prior cholecystectomy, check for the presence of a choledochoduodenal fistula about an inch above the papilla. This is the weakest point in the extrahepatic bile duct wall, which is sometimes perforated when surgeons probe the bile duct with dilators during cholecystectomy. The surgeon thinks that he or she has passed the probe through the papilla into the duodenum, but, in fact, a suprapapillary fistula (**Fig. 1**) has been created instead. Surgically created choledochoduodenal anastomoses are usually found in the duodenal bulb (D1). As they are often large, cholangiography through these openings may require occluding them first with a balloon catheter, then injecting contrast under pressure (occlusion cholangiography). Duodenal diverticula frequently involve the main papilla, significantly altering the axis of the bile duct, and sometimes complicating cannulation (**Fig. 2**). I still get referrals from community endoscopists who abandon ERCP as soon as they see the papilla anywhere in the vicinity of a diverticulum; however, in practice, most papillas in and around duodenal diverticula can be cannulated with minor modifications to standard technique. The "danger" of diverticula is their thin wall and the risk of perforation from repeated unsuccessful instrumentation. Adjunctive techniques, especially stenting the PD first (**Fig. 3**), can

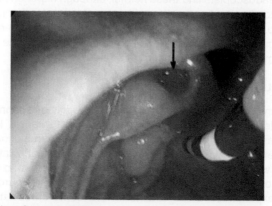

Fig. 1. Suprapapillary fistula (*arrow*).

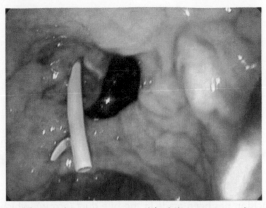

Fig. 2. Main papilla after sphincterotomy with biliary stent placement, showing its relationship to a periampullary diverticulum.

significantly increase the safety and success of biliary cannulation and therapy in this setting. Great care must be taken when using a needle knife near or within a diverticulum; however, with a relaxed patient and a steady hand, small, precise incisions can be made safely (**Fig. 4**). The increasing trend toward monitored anesthesia care and general anesthesia for ERCP has undoubtedly led to more successful procedures.[6] Trying to cannulate a tiny target in an agitated, retching, inadequately sedated patient is a miserable experience for all concerned, and a challenge even for an expert. Leaving aside the current debate about who should be allowed to administer anesthesia for endoscopy, there is no doubt that anesthesia-assisted ERCP is here to stay.

If we look at the "normal" duodenal papilla using the duodenoscope, the axis of the bile duct should be in the 11 o'clock position, while the PD courses "backward" and a little to the right (the 3 o'clock position) (**Fig. 5**). When attempting to access the bile duct with a cannula, the tip should be used to gently probe the papilla in the expected

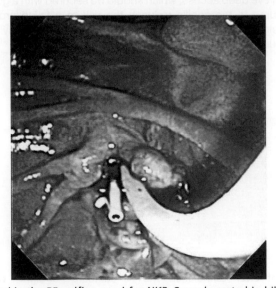

Fig. 3. Stent seated in the PD orifice, used for NKP. Cannula seated in bile duct.

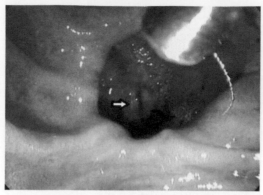

Fig. 4. Small NKP incision has been made in the bile duct (*arrow*), which is running up the back wall of a periampullary diverticulum.

direction. If an orifice is not visible, there are usually clues to its whereabouts in the fine surface anatomy. With a straight catheter, biliary cannulation requires coming at the papilla from below; with a papillotome one has the advantage of being able to vary the tip angulation by tightening or relaxing the cutting wire. Gentle lifting using the elevator (or "bridge") and/or pulling the endoscope back a little will often "seat" the catheter in the biliary opening; however, if a papillotome is being used, in a "bowed" configuration, the upward angle of the tip may actually impede deep cannulation by impacting on the "roof" of the duct. The "trick" to advancing the catheter at this point is to reduce the tip angulation by a small amount (relax the cutting wire), which brings it into line with the bile duct axis (**Fig. 6**). This makes the process sound easy, which it is frequently not.

A "floppy" papilla or one in an anatomically unfavorable orientation (eg, within a diverticulum) requires experimentation with different cannulation angles and sometimes one or more adjunctive techniques (including some of those described later in this article) to achieve deep access, which should be secured with a guide wire. Avoiding repeated trauma to the papilla reduces the risk of a failed procedure and the subsequent development of post-ERCP pancreatitis. Also, the early recognition that NKP may be required for access is important.

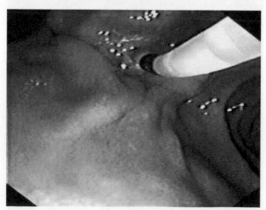

Fig. 5. A view of ERCP cannulation with a standard "straight" catheter (ie, not a papillotome).

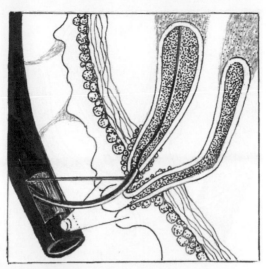

Fig. 6. Biliary sphincterotomy after guide wire access.

GUIDE WIRE–ASSISTED CANNULATION

The technique of leading with a guide wire can be very helpful. A short length of guide wire (eg, 1 cm) is advanced beyond the tip of the catheter and used to gently probe in the expected axis of the desired duct. A 0.021-inch-diameter or 0.025-inch-diameter coated guide wire works best. If the guide wire can be advanced deep into the duct, the catheter can then be advanced over it. Care must be taken not to force the wire: even wires with a hydrophilic coating can be traumatic. Assistants need to be taught to push the wire gently, and withdraw if they see the catheter being pushed backward. A wire seen to be going in an unexpected direction (on fluoroscopy) is probably misplaced, and should be withdrawn immediately. If the guide wire tip loops in the duct, this adds a measure of safety to the procedure. Any resistance to the passage of the wire should raise concern for the appropriateness of its placement. This is especially true in the PD, where is it is easy to perforate a small side branch. This often results in post-ERCP pancreatitis, presumably from local extravasation of pancreatic juice into the parenchyma. The key to therapeutic ERCP is not only gaining access to the duct of choice, but maintaining it. There are few experiences in endoscopy more frustrating than having obtained a cholangiogram or pancreatogram, then losing access. Inexperienced assistants often fail to appreciate how easily the guide wire can be pulled out. Plenty of practice with wire exchanges (eg, for stent placement) usually solves this problem, as it teaches the assistant fine control of guide wire insertion and withdrawal.

GUIDE WIRE–ASSISTED BILIARY ACCESS

Guide wires may also be used to assist biliary cannulation and sphincterotomy. If the cannula tip repeatedly enters the PD, placing a guide wire in the duct serves 2 potential purposes. First, with the PD orifice identified and partially occluded by the wire, it becomes easier to work out where the bile duct orifice should be. Modern duodenoscope instrument channels are wide enough to accommodate a wire placed in the PD and a papillotome or other catheter advanced alongside for biliary access (**Fig. 7**). The second function of the guide wire is to provide orientation for a needle knife or other

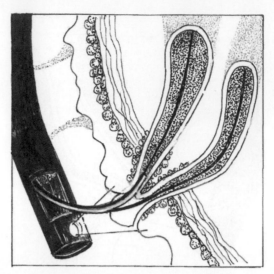

Fig. 7. Wire-assisted biliary cannulation (guide wire in main PD).

precutting device; with the PD axis clearly identified, it is straightforward to direct the incision upward (cephalad) and away from the pancreas. A note of caution is appropriate here, however. Although the length of the wire typically has an insulated coating, the very tip, which is deep within the PD, may not. At least theoretically, this may provide a conduit for *induced current,* resulting from adjacent electrocautery, to be transmitted into the PD, risking ductal injury and pancreatitis. I personally have not seen this complication, but the (albeit small) risk of it has discouraged me from using the technique. Instead, I prefer to use the guide wire in the PD to place a small-caliber (typically a 5-Fr gauge, single pigtail, single flanged) plastic stent, over which I can perform precut papillotomy (**Fig. 8**). This stent is left at the end of the procedure to provide prophylaxis against post-ERCP pancreatitis.[7] Most such stents work their way out into the duodenum within 3 to 7 days, passing spontaneously in the stool. The pigtail left in the duodenum prevents inward migration, a complication well worth avoiding.

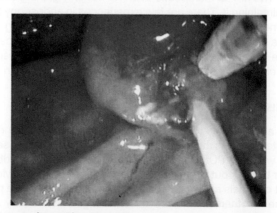

Fig. 8. NKP down on to ("over") a PD stent.

Precut (Access) or NKP

Historically, precut papillotomy has referred to cutting procedures from the outside of the papilla, when deep (usually biliary) access cannot be obtained. These days, the term is almost synonymous with NKP: both imply the use of so-called "free-hand" incision of the papillary roof or septum with a bare wire, emerging from a plastic sheath, through which current is passed (**Fig. 9**). It is a less-controlled "cut" than a standard papillotomy using a "pull" papillotome. NKP has long had the reputation of being a procedure for experts only, in part because of its potential for causing injury, including bleeding, perforation, and pancreatitis. Historically, NKP has been associated with a higher risk of post-ERCP pancreatitis (PEP) than seen with standard papillotomy, often quoted as approximately 15%.[8] This is unfair to the technique, however, which is often used after repeated unsuccessful cannulation attempts that are probably responsible for the pancreatitis. Experts typically use the NKP technique early in the procedure, recognizing the risks of repeat unsuccessful instrumentations of the papilla. As a result, they often report *lower* than standard PEP rates for needle knife procedures. Some exponents of NKP prefer to cut "down" on to the papillary fold, creating a fistula (fistulotomy), which is extended caudad, toward the ampulla. A "downward" cut can also be made on to a previously placed pancreatic stent or guide wire seated deep in the PD. It is probably safer to make a precut in a cephalad ("upward") direction, however (ie, away from the pancreas) (**Fig. 10**).

Safe NKP requires an appreciation of the papillary anatomy, and the likely axis of the bile duct. The bile duct typically courses just a few millimeters below the surface, so downward pressure risks penetrating the back wall of the duct and causing a local perforation. Pressure should *never* be used when performing NKP: the comparison between the needle knife catheter and a hot table knife cutting through butter is appropriate. One of the great exponents of NKP, Professor Kees Huibregtse, of Amsterdam, used to compare NKP technique to using a paint brush: the aim should be to make light strokes across the surface while applying current. The lack of a satisfactory locking mechanism on most commercially available needle knives makes precise depth control difficult. Cuts of not more than 2-mm to 3-mm depth at a time are the goal. With patience, the choledochus (common bile duct) can be dissected free from its surroundings. The choledochus has a white ("Mother of Pearl") luster that distinguishes it from surrounding tissue (**Fig. 11**). Once the structure is exposed, a small incision is made to access the lumen; success is usually indicated by a trickle of bile from this opening. I prefer to extend the initial incision with a standard papillotome,

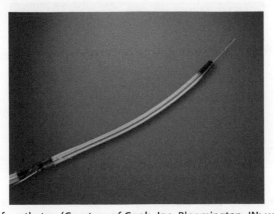

Fig. 9. Needle knife catheter. (*Courtesy of* Cook, Inc, Bloomington, IN; with permission.)

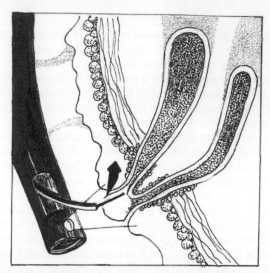

Fig. 10. Free-hand NKP in a cephalad direction. The "lip" of the biliary orifice will be lifted to move the needle tip away from the PD orifice. In expert hands this is a safe maneuver, but it is safer to stent the PD orifice first.

which is inserted through the fistula. Sometimes it is necessary to probe this opening with a guide wire to establish deep cannulation. With the guide wire in place, the bile duct can be further "de-roofed" in a safe fashion. If a fistulotomy is performed, the incision can be extended upward (cephalad) using the needle knife, or a guide wire can be advanced down the duct and out through the papilla. This guide wire can then be grasped with a basket or snare catheter and pulled up through the instrument channel of the scope, establishing a way for a standard papillotome to get seated across the papilla to perform a standard "cut."

ELECTROCAUTERY WITH THE NEEDLE KNIFE

Endoscopists as a group tend to have a rather rudimentary understanding of the physics of electrocautery.[9] The current density at the tip of the needle knife wire is

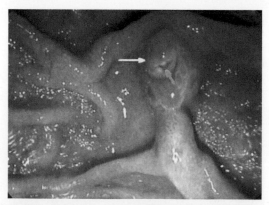

Fig. 11. Choledochus (bile duct) exposed by NKP (*yellow arrow* = bile duct dissected partially free; *green arrow* = needle knife fistula into bile duct).

inversely related to the square of the length in contact with tissue, and to the cube of the area. If, as is usual, only the tip of the needle knife is in contact with tissue, the *current density* at that point is huge. At standard electrocautery settings for endoscopic sphincterotomy, the needle knife provides a very rapid cut with minimal coagulation of blood vessels, so some bleeding is typical. Beginners should experiment with lower power settings, and use the minimum needed to achieve the desired effect. Pressure on the tissue being incised is unnecessary and should be avoided, as this invites a deeper-than-intended cut and risks perforation. The needle knife should always be visible to the endoscopist: "blind" cutting within the bile duct or (especially) the PD invites trouble, and should be avoided.

FISTULOTOMY

Making a puncture into a dilated bile duct is called a fistulotomy. When the bile duct is very dilated, the papillary fold is usually prominent, and it is rarely difficult to identify a safe spot for needle knife incision. An advantage of fistulotomy is that it keeps the operator at a distance from the pancreas; however, if the duodenal papilla cannot be traversed, fistulotomy can leave a distal bile duct "sump" in which sludge and stones can form. A cystic dilatation of the distal choledochus, a choledochocele (Type III choledochal cyst), is a particularly inviting target for fistulotomy (**Figs. 12** and **13**). If there is any doubt about the nature of this pear-shaped structure protruding into the lumen of the duodenum where the normal papilla should be, EUS is an elegant way to confirm the diagnosis.

NKP: FOR EXPERTS ONLY?

It is the author's that belief that rather than being a procedure for experts only, NKP should be taught to all endoscopists intending to perform therapeutic ERCP on a regular basis. To achieve a cannulation rate close to 100%, it is necessary to be adept at NKP. Typically, NKP is reserved for therapeutic indications, but experts can and do use it periodically for difficult diagnostic access. NKP requires supervised training and experience: it is not a procedure that can or should be self-taught. How many NKPs should a trainee do before doing it unsupervised? There are no widely accepted numbers representing a threshold for competence, in part because the difficulty of the procedure

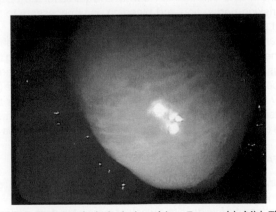

Fig. 12. Choledochocele (Type III choledochal cyst) in a 7-year-old child. This cystic structure occupies the expected location of the main duodenal papilla in the second part of duodenum.

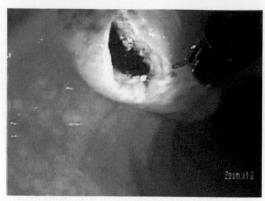

Fig. 13. Fistulotomy with extension of the opening reveals that the choledochocele is occupied by a large pigmented stone.

depends on the setting and the indication. NKP is relatively safe when dealing with dilated bile ducts in the elderly, but considerably more risky when attempting to access small (nondilated) ducts in younger patients. Probably the commonest reason for failure to access the bile duct by NKP is veering off its axis. Once a cut is started in the wrong place, the papillary anatomy becomes distorted, and it can be difficult to find one's way back. Marking the anticipated axis of the duct with tiny burns from the tip of the needle knife is one way to keep on track. It is surprising that (to the best of my knowledge) no accessory maker has yet developed a marker pen on the tip of a catheter for this purpose. The problem of identifying the local anatomy is often compounded by bleeding; the needle knife cuts so quickly that little vessel cautery occurs. The base of the incision often becomes obscured by blood. Repeated washing is usually necessary to maintain a satisfactory view. I like to use a dilute solution of epinephrine for these washes, as I believe, without any scientific proof, that this reduces capillary oozing. How far cephalad the cut can safely be extended depends on the size of the papilla, and the courage of the endoscopist; however, the upper limit in most cases should be where the papillary mound meets the duodenal wall (or the so-called "hooding fold"). It is wise to limit the extent of the needle knife incision to what is required for the job at hand. Creating a huge opening, risking perforation and bleeding, is unnecessary to retrieve a 1-cm-diameter bile duct stone, for example.

I like to add a transverse cut at the top of my NKPs to create a "T" shape. This allows the upper end of the vertical incision to be spread apart, often revealing the shiny surface of the choledochus. When the bile duct has been chronically obstructed, as in malignant jaundice, its wall becomes thickened and takes on a waxy appearance (**Fig. 14**). Cutting through this waxy surface with the needle knife takes a little longer than the typical, lightning-fast incision it makes through normal tissue. It takes some experience to recognize the bile duct in this setting and adjust the cutting technique accordingly.

OPTIONS AFTER FAILED ENDOSCOPIC BILE DUCT ACCESS

What should be done if access to the bile duct cannot be obtained? Until relatively recently, it was not uncommon for NKP to fail to expose the bile duct; patients would be brought back for a second attempt a few days to a week or more later, if the clinical situation would allow such delay. Not infrequently, the biliary fistula would be obvious at this second attempt, after local edema from the initial instrumentation had settled. Severely ill patients

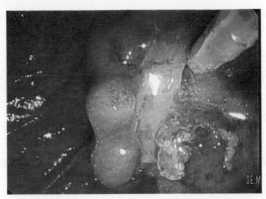

Fig. 14. The waxy ("Mother of Pearl") appearance of the bile duct in chronic obstruction (after NKP).

with acute cholangitis who fail endoscopic drainage require urgent biliary decompression, however, which is usually achieved by interventional radiology (eg, percutaneous biliary drain). The presence of a percutaneous biliary catheter offers the possibility of a combined radiologic-endoscopic procedure to establish access through the papilla for therapeutic procedures.[10] If a guide wire can be negotiated "downward" through the papilla into the duodenum, its end can be grasped with a basket catheter or snare and the wire pulled up through the instrument channel. Provided that it is sufficiently long (eg, 450 cm), the guide wire can then be used in the standard fashion to advance accessories down into the duodenum for sphincterotomy, stenting, and so forth. Combined procedures were common during the 1990s, and used too often as an alternative to skill at selective biliary cannulation. In addition to being cumbersome and time-consuming, however, combined radiologic-endoscopic procedures were shown to increase morbidity and hospital stay. In current ERCP practice, with the various adjunctive techniques that have been developed to improve access, combined procedures should be a rarity; however, they remain useful when access to the bile duct is limited by malignancy or atypical anatomy. Another option, a detailed description of which is beyond the scope of this review, is EUS-assisted biliary access.[11] An obstructed and inaccessible bile duct or PD identified by EUS can often be punctured using an EUS aspirating needle, a ductogram obtained, and a guide wire passed (cephalad or caudad) to establish biliary access for therapeutic procedures, such as stenting. This is not without risk, as the pioneers of EUS-assisted biliary and PD access have discovered. In part, the complications of these EUS techniques relate to the lack of specialized tools to establish and maintain the fistula that is created by needle puncture. Several endoscopic accessory companies are in the process developing such tools, which will render EUS-assisted biliary and pancreatic endotherapy easier and therefore more widely available.

MODIFICATIONS OF STANDARD BILIARY ACCESS TECHNIQUES
The Goff Technique (Trans-Septal Sphincterotomy)

A variant of the standard technique of papillotomy involved positioning the papillotome in the PD and cutting cephalad, through the septum separating the pancreatic and bile ducts. This transpancreatic technique was first pioneered by a US gastroenterologist, and is often referred to as the Goff Technique.[12] Dr Goff found no increase in PEP with this technique, which is usually used when bile duct cannulation has been unsuccessful and the papillotome repeatedly enters the PD instead.

Shark-Fin Papillotomy

The cutting wire on the so-called shark-fin papillotome is applied to the wall of the papillary fold, and the cut made with inward pressure (**Fig. 15**). Few modern ERCP endoscopists have ever used one, as NKP has largely replaced this somewhat cumbersome approach.

Endoscopic Ampullectomy/Papillectomy

Removing the duodenal papilla ("ampulla") will expose the orifices of the bile duct and PD (**Fig. 16**). Some investigators have recommended this approach when standard cannulation techniques have been unsuccessful.[13] Unless there is another reason to remove the papilla (eg, ampullary adenoma), I consider this to be a rather aggressive and somewhat risky way to deal with failed access. If this procedure is used, it is very important to place a prophylactic PD stent, otherwise post-ERCP pancreatitis is likely to follow.

Suprapapillary Blunt Dissection

In suprapapillary blunt dissection, a linear needle knife cut is made in the mucosa overlying the papillary fold. Then, a small ball of cotton held by endoscopic forceps is used for blunt dissection down to the bile duct, which is then opened with the needle knife. Although there have been publications regarding this approach,[14] it has yet to "catch on."

Endoscopic Scissors

Cutting devices that look like scissors have been used to deroof the papilla as a way to achieve biliary access. There are limited data on this technique[15]; endoscopic scissors have not gained popularity.

BILIARY ACCESS IN THE SETTING OF DIFFICULT ANATOMY
Post-Billroth II Gastrectomy Cannulation

Since the introduction of H2-blockers, then proton pump inhibitors, and the discovery of Helicobacter's role in duodenal ulceration, surgery for gastric and duodenal ulcer

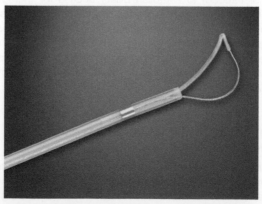

Fig. 15. Shark-fin papillotome. (*Courtesy of* Cook, Inc, Bloomington, IN; with permission.)

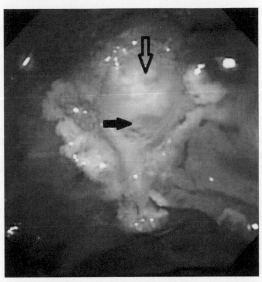

Fig. 16. Duodenal wall immediately following endoscopic (snare) ampullectomy (*open arrow* = bile duct opening; *closed arrow* = PD opening).

has become quite uncommon; however, there are still many patients in the community who had surgical rearrangement of their upper GI tract before effective pharmacologic interventions came along. The classic Billroth-II gastrectomy removes the gastric antrum and creates a gastroenterostomy. To reach the main duodenal papilla to perform ERCP, the duodenoscope has to be passed up the afferent limb of small bowel anastomosis. The papilla has to be approached from "below." The flexibility of modern duodenoscopes has increased the success rate for ERCP in this setting, and most experienced endoscopists are comfortable undertaking this procedure. This is one situation in which a straight catheter can be helpful, as from below it is often a "straight shot" into the bile duct using one. Although modified "Billroth-II" papillotomes are available, in my experience they rarely make the job easy. I prefer to start with a standard papillotome and guide wire. Not infrequently, the catheter can be partially or completely rotated into a standard orientation to perform biliary sphincterotomy. Often, it is easier to place a biliary or pancreatic stent then cut down over it with a needle knife. In cases of particular difficulty for access, a combined radiologic-endoscopic approach (a so-called "rendezvous procedure") can be helpful.

ERCP After Bariatric (Weight Loss) Surgery

The current epidemic of obesity in Western countries has resulted in ever-increasing numbers of patients undergoing surgical rearrangement of the GI tract for weight loss. The current most popular bariatric surgery involved creating a long Roux-type limb of small intestine, such that the duodenal papilla is out of reach of the standard duodenoscope. The papilla can be reached in many cases with an enteroscope, but without an "elevator," the instrument is much less versatile than the standard duodenoscope. Also, there are far fewer ERCP accessories available for use through an enteroscope.[16] The alternative approach is laparoscopic-assisted ERCP: a laparoscopic "port" is created into the antrum of the stomach that provides a "short cut" to the papilla for ERCP.[17] The duodenoscope is passed through the laparoscope, bypassing the mouth and esophagus. Another option is to create a percutaneous track into the stomach for endoscopic access (a modification of the standard percutaneous endoscopic gastrostomy procedure). The tract has to be allowed to mature for at least 4 to 6 weeks before it can be used, so this approach is not suitable for patients needing urgent ERCP procedures.

EUS-Guided Biliary and Pancreatic Ductal Access

A detailed discussion of the evolving field of EUS-guided therapeutics is beyond the scope of this review, but using this valuable imaging technique, otherwise endoscopically inaccessible bile ducts and PDs can be entered using fine-needle catheters to accomplish both diagnostic and therapeutic procedures (**Fig. 17**). These applications are in their infancy; wider use of them awaits a new generation of accessories for creating fistulas across the stomach and duodenal walls, and maintaining patency thereafter.

Minor Duodenal Papilla Access

When investigating and treating the anatomic variant of pancreas divisum, the minor papilla has to be accessed for dorsal duct pancreatography. This is a tiny target and requires particular skill to identify and cannulate, sometimes after an injection of a synthetic form of the hormone, secretin, to enhance the anatomy.[18] Historically, a cannula with a short metal tip (Cremer catheter, Cook, Inc., Winston-Salem, NC) has been the preferred instrument for probing the minor papilla, but this tip can be traumatic. I prefer to use a small-caliber papillotome with a 0.021-inch or 0.025-inch guide wire. Typically, minor papillotomy is performed using NKP over a small-caliber stent placed in the orifice (**Fig. 18**).

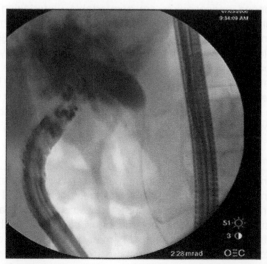

Fig. 17. EUS-assisted biliary access. This cholangiogram was obtained after EUS-guided puncture of the obstructed bile duct from the duodenal bulb. (*Courtesy of* Dr Jason Conway, MD, Wake Forest University Baptist Medical Center, Winston-Salem, NC.)

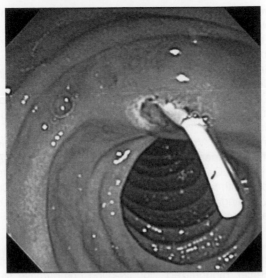

Fig. 18. Minor papillotomy (NKP) over a stent placed in the dorsal PD (to treat symptomatic pancreas divisum).

ACKNOWLEDGMENTS

The author thanks Ann Hauman of Beaufort, NC, for creating the excellent line drawings for this review.

REFERENCES

1. Freeman ML, Guda NM. ERCP cannulation: a review of reported techniques. Gastrointest Endosc 2005;61(1):112–25.
2. Schutz SM, Abbott RM. Grading ERCPs by degree of difficulty: a new concept to produce more meaningful outcome data. Gastrointest Endosc 2000;51:535–9.
3. Rossos PG, Kortan P, Haber G. Selective common bile duct cannulation can be simplified by the use of a standard papillotome. Gastrointest Endosc 1993;39: 67–9.
4. Igarashi Y, Tada T, Shimura J, et al. A new cannula with a flexible tip (Swing Tip) may improve the success rate of endoscopic retrograde cholangiopancreatography. Endoscopy 2002;34:628–31.
5. Deviere J. Pancreatic stents. Gastrointest Endosc Clin N Am 2011;21(3):499–510.
6. Mehta PP, Vargo JJ, Dumot JA, et al. Does anesthesiologist-directed sedation for ERCP improve deep cannulation and complication rates? Dig Dis Sci 2001;56(7): 2185–90.
7. Arain MA, Freeman ML. Pancreatic endoscopic retrograde cholangiopancreatography. Endoscopy 2011;43(1):47–53.
8. Dowsett JF, Polydorou AA, Vaira D, et al. Needle knife papillotomy: how safe and how effective? Gut 1990;31:905–90.
9. Siegal JH, Bon Zvi JS, Pillano W. The needle knife: a valuable tool in diagnostic and therapeutic ERCP. Gastrointest Endosc 1989;35(6):499–503.
10. Wayman J, Mansfield JC, Matthewson K, et al. Combined percutaneous and endoscopic procedures for bile duct obstruction: simultaneous and delayed techniques compared. Hepatogastroenterology 2003;50(52):915–8.

11. Chavilitdhamrong D, Dragonov PV. Endoscopic ultrasound-guided biliary drainage [review]. World J Gastroenterol 2012;18(6):491–7.
12. Goff JS. Long term experience with the transpancreatic sphincter precut approach to biliary sphincterotomy. Gastrointest Endosc 1999;50:642–5.
13. Wong RF, DiSario JA. Approaches to endoscopic ampullectomy. Curr Opin Gastroenterol 2004;20(5):460–7.
14. Hashiba K, D'Assuncao MA, Armelli S, et al. Endoscopic suprapapillary dissection of the common bile duct in cases of difficult cannulation: a pilot study. Endoscopy 2004;36:317–21.
15. Heiss FW, Cimis RS Jr, MacMillan FP Jr. Biliary sphincter scissors for pre-cut access: preliminary experience. Gastrointest Endosc 2002;55:719–22.
16. Monkemuller K, Fry LC, Bellutti M, et al. ERCP with the double balloon enteroscope in patients with roux-en Y anastomosis. Surg Endosc 2009;23:1961–7.
17. Schreiner MA, Chang L, Gluck M, et al. Laparoscopy-assisted versus balloon enteroscopy assisted ERCP in bariatric post Roux-en Y bypass patients. Gastrointest Endosc 2012;75:748–56.
18. Devereaux BM, Fein S, Purich E, et al. A new synthetic porcine secretin for facilitation of cannulation of the dorsal duct at ERCP in patients with pancreas divisum: a multicenter, randomized, double-blind comparative study. Gastrointest Endosc 2003;57(6):643–7.

Endoscopic Retrograde Cholangiopancreatography for Stone Burden in the Bile and Pancreatic Ducts

Laura Rosenkranz, MD*, Sandeep N. Patel, DO

KEYWORDS

- Endoscopic retrograde cholangiopancreatography • Cholangioscopy
- Bile duct stones • Pancreatic duct stones

KEY POINTS

- Stones in the bile duct and pancreatic duct are entities that plague hundreds of thousands of patients worldwide every year.
- Symptoms can be mild (pain) to life threatening (cholangitis, severe acute pancreatitis). In the last few decades, management of these stones has transitioned from exclusively surgical to now predominantly endoscopic techniques.
- This article reviews the evolution of endoscopic techniques used in the management of stones in the common bile duct and pancreatic duct.

BILE DUCT STONES

Conventional Endoscopic Therapies

The management of common bile duct (CBD) stones was predominantly surgical for almost 100 years. The introduction of endoscopic sphincterotomy (ES) by Classen and Demling[1] and Kawai and colleagues[2] in the early 1970s not only pioneered therapeutic endoscopy but set in motion a shift to its predominant use in the management of biliary stones (**Fig. 1**). ES over the years has become well established as a safe technique, with an overall complication rate of approximately 5%.[3] Additional early developments of tools such as extraction balloons and the Dormia basket led to successful endoscopic removal of bile duct stones in more than 80% of patients.[4]

Demling and colleagues[5] published the first experience of mechanical lithotripsy to fragment difficult stones and thereby facilitate successful removal in 1982. Mechanical

Disclosure: None.
Department of Medicine, University of Texas Health Science Center at San Antonio, 7300 Floyd Curl Drive Mail Code 7878, San Antonio, TX 78229, USA
* Corresponding author.
E-mail address: Rosenkranz@uthscsa.edu

Gastrointest Endoscopy Clin N Am 22 (2012) 435–450
doi:10.1016/j.giec.2012.05.007
1052-5157/12/$ – see front matter © 2012 Elsevier Inc. All rights reserved.

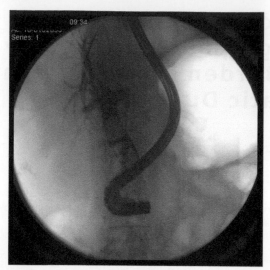

Fig. 1. Fluoroscopic image of large (>2 cm) bile duct stones.

lithotripsy has been shown to be a relatively simple and cost-effective way of frag-menting stones. This modality entails capturing the stone within a basket and then closing it against the metal sleeve of the basket catheter, causing fragmentation of the stone. A variety of both reusable and single-use through-the-scope mechanical lithotripsy devices are available. One of the major potential hazards of stone extraction using a standard plastic-sheathed basket is impaction of stone and basket at the level of the ampulla. In this situation a Soehendra-type "emergency" metal lithotripter sheath is passed over the impacted basket's exposed wires, following cutting off the basket handle and removal of both the duodenoscope and the plastic sheath covering the basket wires. Under fluoroscopic guidance, additional traction is applied resulting in fragmentation of the stones or rupture of the basket wires, facilitating either stone or basket removal. Failure to have available or use this device has led to inad-vertent surgical intervention. Demling's study and other subsequent studies have shown mechanical lithotripsy to improve endoscopic bile duct clearance rates to approximately 90%.

Failure with the aforementioned modalities has been associated with the following clinical situations: (1) stones exceeding 2 cm in size; (2) limited sphincterotomy owing to anatomic constraints (small papilla, periampullary diverticulum); (3) stones proximal to a stricture or in difficult locations (cystic or intrahepatic ducts); and (4) impacted stones. The next 3 sections review the nonconventional methods used to remove diffi-cult bile duct stones, and should be used only when the previously mentioned tech-niques have failed.

Balloon Sphincteroplasty

Endoscopic balloon dilation (EBD, sphincteroplasty) was introduced in 1983 by Staritz and colleagues[6] as an alternative to ES for the treatment of bile stones. EBD refers to the controlled expansion of the sphincter of Oddi with a 4- to 8-mm dilation balloon, usually over 30 seconds to a few minutes. This action facilitates extraction of moderate-sized stones (5–8 mm) from the bile duct using conventional tools such as baskets or balloon catheters; however, this approach frequently requires mechanical lithotripsy for stones larger than 8 mm.[7,8] Two meta-analyses comparing EBD and ES for stone clearance found similar success rates between the two therapies with a decreased rate of pancreatitis in the patients treated with ES.[9,10] Although EBD offers theoretical advantages of a sphincter-preserving alternative to sphincterotomy, serious complications such as severe pancreatitis have brought the safety of this technique into question.[11,12] One multicenter, randomized controlled trial of EBD versus ES was discontinued because of preliminary findings of increased risk of short-term morbidity and death related to pancreatitis in the EBD arm.[13] Alternatively, EBD appears to carry a lower risk of bleeding and perforation, leading to its recommendation for treatment of choledocholithiasis in patients with coagulopathy.[7–13]

In 2003, Ersoz and colleagues[14] introduced a novel approach for the management of difficult stones that has since been termed endoscopic sphincterotomy with large balloon dilation (ESLBD) or endoscopic papillary large balloon dilation (EPLBD). A small sphincterotomy is made followed by a large (10–20 mm) balloon dilation, allowing for extraction of very large CBD stones (**Fig. 2**). The size of the balloon is matched not to exceed that of the distal bile duct, and is inflated with contrast under fluoroscopic guidance until the waist at the level of the sphincter is obliterated. A recent meta-analysis comparing EPLBD with ES for treatment of large stones noted fewer complications in the EPLBD group and decreased need for mechanical lithotripsy.[15] Unlike EBD, EPLBD does not appear to be associated with an increased risk of pancreatitis[16] (**Table 1**). The initial separation of biliary from pancreatic sphincters created by the biliary ES appears to then facilitate a controlled balloon-induced

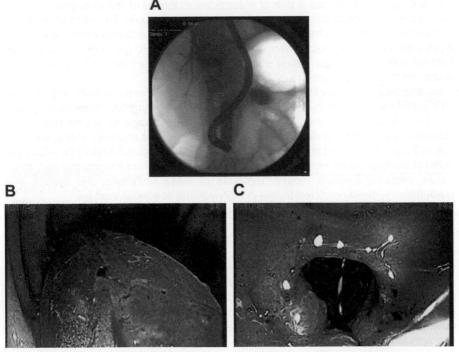

Fig. 2. Endoscopic papillary large balloon dilation (EPLBD). (*A*) Fluoroscopic image of 15-mm balloon dilation of ampulla. (*B*) Endoscopic image of 15-mm balloon dilation of ampulla. (*C*) Large opening of the papillary orifice after EPLBD.

Table 1				
Results of EBD and EPLBD for the treatment of large CBD stones				
Authors	No. of Trials/ Patients	Balloon Size (mm)	Clearance (%)	Complications Overall/Pancreatitis (%)
EBD				
Baron and Harewood[10]	8/552	≤8	94	11/7
Weinberg et al[9]	15/878	8–12	90	10/9
Disario et al[13]	117	≤8	97	18/15
EPLBD				
Feng et al[15]	7/378	12–20	97	6/4
Ersoz et al[14]	58	10–20	89	15/3
Draganov et al[17]	44	10–15	84	7/0

tear away from the pancreatic orifice. EPLBD seeks to combine the advantages of dilation with the safety profile of ES, and has thus far shown promising results in the United States and elsewhere.

Electrohydraulic Lithotripsy

When mechanical lithotripsy and or EPLBD have failed, shock-wave lithotripsy can be used to fragment bile duct stones and thereby facilitate removal. In electrohydraulic lithotripsy (EHL), shock waves are created in a liquid media by the generation of high-voltage sparks across a pair of electrodes at the tip of the EHL probe, which instantaneously evaporates fluid, creating a cavitation bubble. The oscillation of this bubble then forms a mechanical shock wave that subsequently fragments the stone, a process termed the electromechanic effect of EHL. EHL generates considerable thermal energy, which can cause significant bile duct injury and is thus performed under direct visual guidance.

Intraductal shock-wave lithotripsy can be performed under peroral cholangioscopic (POC) guidance currently by 1 of 2 methods. The mother-daughter endoscopic system has been in use since the 1970s and entails the passage of a cholangioscope (daughter) through the working channel of a duodenoscope (mother). This system requires 2 experienced endoscopists to operate the endoscopes. Ultrathin (3.1–3.4 mm) video cholangioscopes with 2-way tip deflection offer excellent imaging but tend to be fragile, requiring frequent repairs. Because of these limitations, this system has predominantly been restricted to use in high-volume academic centers.

The recently developed single-operator catheter-based system (SpyGlass; Boston Scientific, Natick, MA, USA) has gained increasingly widespread popularity since its introduction in 2005. This system uses a 10F (3.3 mm) disposable catheter with 4-way tip deflection and a reusable fiber optic probe. The catheter is passed over a guide wire through the working channel of the duodenoscope, and its 1.2-mm working channel allows for passage of an EHL probe or other tools such as biopsy forceps. Other channels in this catheter allow for passage of the optical probe and simultaneous fluid irrigation and/or aspiration. Whereas the mother-daughter system offers quality video imaging, the catheter-based system offers a slightly more user-friendly platform to perform intraductal lithotripsy.

EHL probes, typically 3F (1 mm) in diameter, are advanced through the working channel of the POC to the level of the stone. A foot pedal is used to activate 1- to 2-second impulses of EHL in 1- to 2-second bursts at energies ranging from 70 to

100 W. Continuous irrigation of saline into the bile duct seems to increase the conductance of the EHL. Repeat applications are performed until desired fragmentation is achieved.

Piraka and colleagues[18] reported their prospective experience with cholangioscopy-guided EHL for the management of difficult bile duct stones in 30 patients. These patients had previously undergone a mean of 3.3 failed attempts at stone extraction using conventional endoscopic techniques. Complete stone clearance was achieved in 81% with a mean of 1.4 sessions of EHL, with 3 minor procedure-related complications. Long-term follow-up (mean 29 months) revealed recurrent stone formation in 18%.

Several other studies have reported favorable results with EHL, and are summarized in **Table 2**.[19–25] EHL appears to be effective in the fragmentation and removal of large bile duct stones in 79% to 98% of cases. Overall complication rates seen with this technique range from 3% to 15%. The potential for major complications (perforation, hemothorax, and bile leak) represent the major obstacle to using this technique. EHL creates a significant amount of thermal effect; considerable caution must be taken to keep the EHL probe in view and off the biliary mucosa to minimize the risk of ductal injury.

Laser Lithotripsy

Laser lithotripsy differs from EHL in that optical rather than electrical energy is used. Both modalities create shock waves in liquid media via creation of a cavitation bubble, which then causes fragmentation of the stone. Laser-induced shock waves theoretically hit biliary stones precisely, with minimal effects to the biliary epithelium. Prolonged direct tissue contact with laser, however, can cause coagulation-induced bile duct injury and thus should also be performed under direct endoscopic visualization. The physical properties and risks of each laser are determined by several factors, namely, wavelength, pulse duration, and energy (**Table 3**). Over the past few decades, many studies have evaluated the efficacy of laser lithotripsy for large bile duct stones.

Endoscopic retrograde laser lithotripsy of refractory bile duct stones was first reported by Lux and colleagues[26] in 1986 using pulsed neodymium:YAG. In 1990 Cotton and colleagues[27] validated this technique as a safe and effective alternative to surgery by successfully clearing large stones in 20 of 25 patients using a coumarin green dye laser under direct endoscopic guidance, without significant morbidity. The initial studies from Europe used rhodamine 6-G dye via 200- to 300-μm diameter probes under both visual cholangioscopic and fluoroscopic guidance with a stone

Table 2
Electrohydraulic lithotripsy for common bile duct stones

Authors	n	Clearance (%)	Complications
Liguory et al[19]	17	94	Hemobilia = 21
Bonnel et al[20]	50	92	Cholangitis = 22
Binmoeller et al[21]	65	98	Pancreatitis = 3
Siegal et al[22]	21	86	Perforation = 3
Yoshimoto et al[23]	31	97	Hemothorax = 1
Adamek et al[24]	46	74	Bile leak = 1
Arya et al[25]	94	90	
Piraka et al[18]	30	81	
Others[a]	138	83	
	n = 492	μ = 89	Total = 51/492 (10%)

[a] Summary of 23 studies with fewer than 15 patients.

Table 3
Physical properties of various lasers used in gastroenterology

Laser	Wavelength (nm)	Depth of Penetration (mm)
Flashlamp-pumped		
Coumarin dye	504	>5
Rhodamine 6-G dye	595	>5
Solid-state		
Neodymium:YAG	1064	5
Holmium:YAG	2140	.5
Gas		
Argon	350	4
CO_2	10600	.1

tissue-detection system. Clearance of stones in these patients refractory to conventional therapies was seen in 80% to 97%, with ensuing morbidity (pancreatitis, hemobilia, cholangitis) in up to 8%.[28–30]

Frequency-doubled double-pulse neodymium:YAG (FREDDY) was developed in the late 1990s in Germany, with the promise of combining the effectiveness of the dye lasers with the safety and low cost of solid-state lasers. FREDDY uses the combination of coumarin green dye (20%) and neodymium:YAG (80%) in succession to synergistically create a high-intensity shock wave directly on the stone. FREDDY laser is delivered through a balloon catheter and monitored fluoroscopically. Studies have shown this modality to be effective in 88% to 92% with a morbidity of up to 23%.[31–33]

Holmium laser is the newest of the lithotrities to be introduced for fragmentation of bile duct stones (**Figs. 3** and **4**). The holmium:YAG laser has a wavelength of 2140 nm, which is very close to the peak absorption of water (1940 nm). These properties are responsible for many of its favorable attributes. One advantage of holmium is that its shock wave is extremely precise in an aqueous medium, because all scatter is absorbed completely by water. The other safety advantage is that holmium's depth of penetration on tissue (0.5 mm) is one-tenth that of the shorter-wavelength lasers and EHL (>5 mm). Holmium has been shown to be safe on porcine biliary epithelium when used in 5-second bursts between 8 and 12 W.[34]

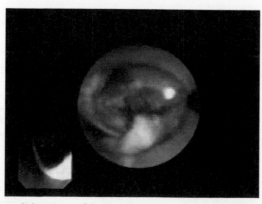

Fig. 3. Successful laser lithotripsy of large CBD stone using SpyGlass-guided holmium:YAG laser lithotripsy.

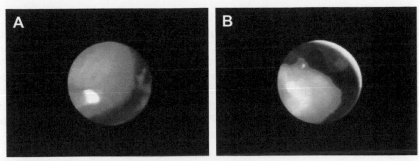

Fig. 4. SpyGlass-guided laser lithotripsy of large CBD stone. (*A*) Laser probe exiting the scope at the 8 o'clock position. (*B*) Successful fragmentation of stone.

Three major studies have evaluated the use of holmium:YAG lithotripsy for fragmentation of large stones. As the delivery vehicle 1 study used a mother-daughter POC[35] whereas the other 2 used single-operator POC.[36,37] These studies showed holmium to be effective in 90% to 100% of patients for stone fragmentation, requiring an average of 1.5 sessions to achieve duct clearance, with complication rates ranging from 4% to 13% (**Table 4**).[35–37]

PANCREATIC DUCT STONES

Chronic pancreatitis (CP) is a multifactorial, complex condition characterized by destruction of pancreatic parenchyma and changes in the ductal structures as an end result of prolonged inflammation. A subgroup of these patients with CP has obstruction of the outflow of pancreatic juice resulting in ductal hypertension, a condition known as obstructive pancreatopathy (OP). OP can lead to abdominal pain of significant severity, episodes of recurrent attacks of acute pancreatitis, and variable degrees of progressive exocrine and endocrine pancreatic insufficiency. Intraductal stones are one of many causes of OP and can be found in 20% to 90% of patients with long-standing disease.[38–40]

Endoscopic removal of pancreatic calculi is technically complex and often requires multiple sessions using various modalities. Successful endoscopic extraction of obstructing pancreatic calculi with partial or complete drainage of secretions has been associated with significant clinical response.[41,42]

Table 4
Results of laser lithotripsy: FREDDY and Holmium:YAG

Authors	n	Clearance (%)	Complications (%)
FREDDY			
Cho et al[31]	52	92	23
Lui et al[32]	30	90	7
Kim et al[33]	17	88	17
Holmium:YAG			
Lee et al[35]	10	90	10
Maydeo et al[36]	60	100	14
Patel et al[37]	69	97	4

Chemistry of Pancreatic Stones

Radiolucent stones are composed of degraded forms of lithostathine-S, an amorphous material solubilized at an acidic pH. These stones cannot be targeted by fluoroscopically guided therapies such as extracorporeal shock-wave lithotripsy (ESWL) and become a therapeutic challenge, specifically when large.[43] The transformation of lithostathine into insoluble peptides creates protein aggregates, some promoting deposition of calcium carbonate. These stones, which fortunately make up a vast majority of stones in the pancreatic duct (PD), are radiopaque and can be visualized and targeted fluoroscopically for ESWL therapy.

Conventional Pancreatic Endotherapy

The aim of pancreatic endotherapy is to alleviate secretory outflow obstruction as guided by the specific etiology of the obstruction. Direct access to the PD, pancreatic sphincterotomy (PS), dilation of associated strictures, stenting, and lithotripsy can be achieved via endoscopic retrograde cholangiopancreatography (ERCP) and pancreatoscopy.

PS may be performed with a pull-type sphincterotome over a guide wire or with a needle-knife incision over a guide wire or a pancreatic stent. Early complications of PS include pancreatitis (2%–7%), bleeding (0%–3%), and perforation (<1%). Late complications, typically sphincter restenosis, occur in fewer than 10% of cases.[44,45]

Small (<5 mm) PD stones can be extracted through the major or minor papilla, as dictated by the presence of standard ductal anatomy or variant anatomy such a pancreas divisum, using routine endoscopic techniques such as PS with balloon or basket extraction. Extraction success rates in these cases range between 50% and 75%.[46]

Stones greater than 5 mm in diameter, stones impacted in the main duct, and those located beyond a stricture require alternative fragmentation methods, such as mechanical lithotripsy, ESWL, EHL, or laser lithotripsy (**Fig. 5**).

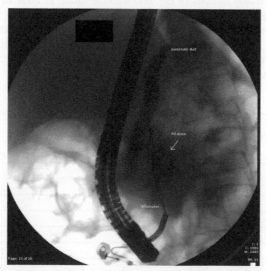

Fig. 5. Attempt to capture a large stone in the head of the pancreas with a mechanical lithotriptor.

Pancreatic Stricture Management

In the setting of CP, PD strictures are typically benign and are related to inflammation, fibrosis, and stone disease. These fibrotic strictures tend to be the rate-limiting step in the stone-extraction process. Stricture dilation methods, including the solitary use of a guide wire with in situ maintenance for 24 hours,[47] the use of balloon or dilating catheters (**Fig. 6**), single or simultaneous placement of multiple plastic endoprostheses,[38,48] and the placement of self-expandable, uncovered Wallstents[49] or fully covered metal stents,[50–52] have all been reported with variable rates of stricture resolution. Stricture resolution allows for the passage of bulky endoscopic devices such as mechanical lithotripters and pancreatoscopes (to permit EHL or laser), and facilitates fragmentation and extraction of large stones (**Fig. 7**).

Extracorporeal Shock-Wave Lithotripsy

The incorporation of ESWL in the nonsurgical management of pancreatic stones was first introduced by Sauerbruch and colleagues[53] in 1987. ESWL works by creating external shock waves in an aqueous environment, which are then focused on the patient's stone(s) using a 2-dimensional fluoroscopic targeting system. When dealing with radiolucent stones, a strategically placed PD stent can be used as the target for the shock waves. Up to a few thousand shock waves can be delivered in one session. The pulverized stone debris is then removed endoscopically, or occasionally will expel out of the duct spontaneously. Complications associated with ESWL include pancreatitis, abdominal pain, and skin and intra-abdominal trauma. Pancreatitis can occur in 5% of patients who undergo ESWL.[54]

In one of the largest series to date, Tandan and Reddy[55] achieved complete PD clearance with ESWL combined with endotherapy in 76% of their 1006 patients. These outcomes were accomplished within 3 ESWL sessions in 96% of the cases. Short-term pain relief was seen in 84%. A large retrospective study involving 11 centers and 555 patients in Japan reported complete PD clearance in 73% with a mean of 5 ESWL sessions with and without endoscopic therapy. Pain relief was experienced

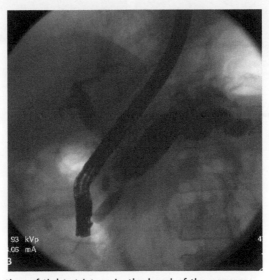

Fig. 6. Balloon dilation of tight stricture in the head of the pancreas.

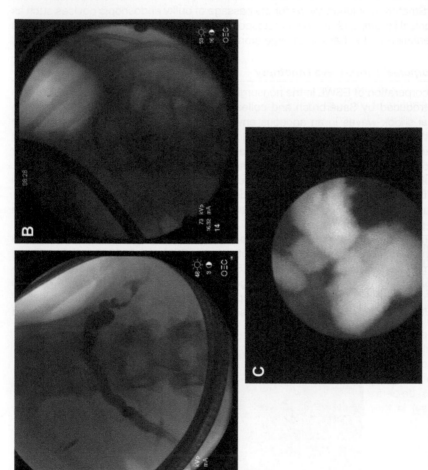

Fig. 7. (A) Pancreatogram revealing 2 large stones in the tail of the pancreas. (B) Passage of the catheter-based POC (SpyGlass) to the tail of the pancreas. (C) Fragmentation of the PD stone(s) with SpyGlass-guided laser lithotripsy.

by 91% immediately. Recurrent stone disease occurred in 22% at 2 years.[55] Other studies using ESWL with and without complementary endoscopic therapy show similar results, and are summarized in **Table 5**. PD clearance rates range from 59% to 74% with this multimodality approach. Short-term pain relief is achieved in 48% to 91% of the patients with complete or partial duct clearance.[54–61]

Intraductal Lithotripsy

Intraductal pancreatic lithotripsy using laser or EHL has the theoretical advantage over ESWL in being a single-step procedure, with fragmentation and removal of pancreatic stones being accomplished in one session. EHL and laser lithotripsy are performed with probes under direct visualization via a pancreatoscope introduced through the working channel of the duodenoscope. Passage of these 3.4-mm scopes (video- or catheter-based) to the level of the stone can be difficult when encountering impacted stones in the pancreatic head, tight strictures, and/or tortuous ducts. Aggressive stricture management with balloon dilation or large-caliber stenting may be a necessity. Data regarding EHL and laser lithotripsy of PD stones is limited. A recent study by Shah and colleagues[62] evaluated the use of holmium:YAG laser lithotripsy in 28 CP patients with large stone burdens. Technical success and complete stone clearance was achieved in 97% and 86% of patients, respectively, in a median of 1 session (range 1–6). Clinical success, defined as a 50% reduction in opiate use, pain scores, or hospitalizations, was achieved in 97%.

Complications of Pancreatic Endotherapy

Conventional pancreatic endotherapy in CP patients with OP is generally well tolerated. The overall reported risk of acute pancreatitis with PD manipulation is 10% to 15%, with most cases successfully managed conservatively. PS is associated with a higher risk of hemorrhage and perforation than is biliary sphincterotomy. Pancreatic duct stenting for prophylactic (to minimize the risk of ERCP-related pancreatitis) or therapeutic (following dilation or other treatment of ductal strictures) purposes may be complicated by pain, stent-induced ductal abnormalities, stent occlusion, proximal or distal stent migration, perforation, and sepsis.[63–68] Mechanical lithotripsy for PD stones carries a markedly increased risk of complications (basket entrapment, fracture, pancreatitis, pancreatic leaks) when compared with lithotripsy for biliary stones, and must be performed with care.[69] The major risk of EHL (and to a lesser degree laser lithotripsy) in the pancreas is heat-induced injury to the PD from direct contact.

Table 5
Extracorporeal shock-wave lithotripsy for PD stones

Authors	n	Complete Clearance (%)	Pain Relief (%)
Delhaye et al[56]	123	59	85
Kozarek et al[57]	40	—	80
Costamagna et al[58]	35	74	72
Tandan and Reddy[55]	1006	76	84
Farnbacher et al[59]	125	64	48
Adamek et al[60]	80	—	76
Lawrence et al[61]	30	58	60
Inui et al[54]	555	73	91

Perforation in this situation can occur in 1% of patients while overall complications, including pancreatitis and bleeding, occur in up to 25%.[62]

SUMMARY

Before the introduction of ESWL in 1989, surgery was the sole alternative for endo-scopically nonremovable PD stones, with success reported in 85% of patients.[70] Although pain-relief outcomes achieved via endoscopic pancreatic drainage in comparison with pancreaticojejunostomy suggested more durable response with surgery (75% in the surgical group versus 32% in the endoscopic therapy group),[71] the debate regarding therapeutic superiority continues, as limitations were identified in the study design. In general, endotherapy is preferred as the initial line of therapy with surgery reserved for those patients in whom endoscopy fails to provide expected outcomes.

Endoscopic management of OP caused by stones, when tailored to selected patients, has potential for distinct clinical benefits but often requires multiple modalities and adjunctive therapies (including ESWL) to accomplish desired outcomes. Further controlled studies, comparing different technologies and therapeutic modalities, although difficult to design and execute in these diverse patients, will continue to provide further insight into the optimal management of this complex pathologic pattern.

ACKNOWLEDGMENTS

Special thanks to Glenn W.W. Gross, MD and John Vizuete for their invaluable contributions to this article.

REFERENCES

1. Classen M, Demling L. Endoskopische Sphincterotomie der Papilla Vateri und Steinextraktion aus dem Ductus Choledochus. Dtsch Med Wochenschr 1974; 99:469 [in German].
2. Kawai K, Akasaka Y, Murakami I, et al. Endoscopic sphincterotomy of the ampulla of Vater. Gastrointest Endosc 1974;20:148.
3. Freeman ML, Nelson DB, Sherman S, et al. Complications of endoscopic biliary sphincterotomy. N Engl J Med 1996;335:909.
4. Cotton PB. Non-operative removal of bile duct stones by duodenoscopic sphinc-terotomy. Br J Surg 1980;67:1.
5. Demling L, Seuberth K, Riemann JF. A mechanical lithotripter. Endoscopy 1982; 14:100.
6. Staritz M, Ewe K, Meyer zum Buschenfelde KH. Endoscopic papillary dilatation, a possible alternative to endoscopic papillotomy. Lancet 1982;1:1306–7.
7. Bergman J, Rauws E, Fockens P, et al. Randomised trial of endoscopic balloon dilation versus endoscopic sphincterotomy for removal of bile duct stones. Lancet 1997;349:1124.
8. MacMathuna P, White P, Clarke E, et al. Endoscopic balloon sphincteroplasty (papillary dilation) for bile duct stones: efficacy, safety, and follow-up in 100 patients. Gastrointest Endosc 1995;42:468.
9. Weinberg BM, Shindy W, Lo S. Endoscopic balloon sphincter dilation (sphincter-oplasty) versus sphincterotomy for common bile duct stones. Cochrane Data-base Syst Rev 2006;4:CD004890.
10. Baron TH, Harewood GC. Endoscopic balloon dilation of the biliary sphincter compared to endoscopic biliary sphincterotomy for removal of common bile

duct stones during ERCP: a meta-analysis of randomized, controlled trials. Am J Gastroenterol 2004;99:1455.

11. Fujita N, Maguchi H, Komatsu Y, et al. Endoscopic sphincterotomy and endoscopic papillary balloon dilation for bile duct stones: a prospective randomized controlled multicenter study. Gastrointest Endosc 2003;57:151–5.

12. Freeman M, DiSario J, Nelson DB, et al. Risk factors for post-ERCP pancreatitis: a prospective, multicenter study. Gastrointest Endosc 2001;54:425–34.

13. Disario JA, Freeman ML, Bjorkman DJ, et al. Endoscopic balloon dilation compared with sphincterotomy for extraction of bile duct stones. Gastroenterology 2004;127:1291–9.

14. Ersoz G, Tekesin O, Ozutemiz AO, et al. Biliary sphincterotomy plus dilation with a large balloon for bile duct stones that are difficult to extract. Gastrointest Endosc 2003;57:156.

15. Feng Y, Zhu H, Chen X, et al. Comparison of endoscopic papillary large balloon dilation and endoscopic sphincterotomy for retrieval of choledocholithiasis: a meta-analysis of randomized controlled trials. J Gastroenterol 2012. [Epub ahead of print].

16. Attam R, Freeman ML. Endoscopic papillary large balloon dilation for large common bile duct stones. J Hepatobiliary Pancreat Surg 2009;16:618.

17. Draganov P, Evans W, Fazel A, et al. Large size balloon dilation of the ampulla after biliary Sphincterotomy can facilitate endoscopic extraction of difficult bile duct stones. J Clin Gastroenterol 2009;43:782.

18. Piraka C, Shah R, Awadallah N, et al. Transpapillary cholangioscopy-directed lithotripsy in patients with difficult bile duct stones. Clin Gastroenterol Hepatol 2007; 5:1333.

19. Liguory CL, Lefebvre JF, Bonnel D, et al. Indications for cholangioscopy. Endoscopy 1989;1:341.

20. Bonnel DH, Liguory CL, Cornud FE, et al. Common bile duct and intrahepatic stones: results of transhepatic electrohydraulic lithotripsy in 50 patients. Radiology 1991;180:345.

21. Binmoeller KF, Bruckner F, Soehendra N. Treatment of difficult bile duct stones using mechanical, electrohydraulic, and extracorporeal shock wave lithotripsy. Endoscopy 1993;25:201.

22. Siegal JH, Ben-Zvi JS, Pullano WE. Endoscopic electrohydraulic lithotripsy. Gastrointest Endosc 1990;36:134.

23. Yoshimoto H, Ikeda S, Tanaka M, et al. Choledoscopic electrohydraulic lithotripsy and lithotomy for stones in the common bile duct, intrahepatic ducts and gallbladder. Ann Surg 1989;210:576.

24. Adamek HE, Maier M, Jakobs R, et al. Management of retained bile duct stones: a prospective open trial comparing extracorporeal and intracorporeal lithotripsy. Gastrointest Endosc 1996;44:40.

25. Arya N, Nelles SE, Haber GB, et al. Electrohydraulic lithotripsy in 111 patients: a safe and effective therapy for difficult bile duct stones. Am J Gastroenterol 2004;99:2330.

26. Lux G, Ell CH, Hochberger J, et al. The first successful endoscopic retrograde laser lithotripsy of common bile duct stones in man using a pulsed neodymium-YAG laser. Endoscopy 1986;18:144–5.

27. Cotton P, Kozarek RA, Shapiro RH, et al. Endoscopic laser lithotripsy of large bile duct stones. Gastroenterology 1990;99:1128.

28. Hochberger J, Bayer J, May A, et al. Laser lithotripsy of difficult bile duct stones: results in 60 patients using rhodamine 6G dye laser with optical stone tissue detection system. Gut 1998;43:823.

29. Jakobs R, Pereira-Lima JC, Schuch AW, et al. Endoscopic laser lithotripsy for complicated bile duct stones: is cholangioscopic guidance necessary? Arq Gastroenterol 2007;44:137.

30. Neuhaus H, Hoffman W, Gottlieb K, et al. Endoscopic lithotripsy of bile duct stones using a new laser with automatic stone recognition. Gastrointest Endosc 1994;40:708.

31. Cho YD, Cheon YK, Moon JH, et al. Clinical role of frequency-doubled double-pulsed yttrium aluminum garnet laser technology for removing difficult bile duct stones. Gastrointest Endosc 2009;70:684.

32. Liu F, Jin ZD, Zou DW, et al. Efficacy and safety of endoscopic biliary lithotripsy using FREDDY laser with a radiopaque mark under fluoroscopic guidance. Endoscopy 2011;43:918.

33. Kim TH, Oh HJ, Choi CS, et al. Clinical usefulness of transpapillary removal of common bile duct stones by frequency doubled double pulse Nd:YAG laser. World J Gastroenterol 2008;14:2863.

34. Patel S, Kiker D, Linsteadt J, et al. Holmium: YAG laser safety data on bile duct epithelium in the porcine model [abstract]. Gastrointest Endosc 2009;69:AB258.

35. Lee TY, Cheon YK, Choe WH, et al. Direct cholangioscopy-based holmium laser lithotripsy of difficult bile duct stones by using an ultrathin upper endoscope without a separate biliary irrigating catheter. Photomed Laser Surg 2012;30:31.

36. Maydeo A, Kwek BE, Bhandari S, et al. Single-operator cholangioscopy-guided laser lithotripsy in patients with difficult biliary and pancreatic ductal stones (with videos). Gastrointest Endosc 2011;74:1308.

37. Patel SN, Rosenkranz L, Hooks B, et al. Holmium-YAG laser lithotripsy in the treatment of pancreatico-biliary calculi utilizing peroral single operator cholangioscopy (SpyGlass): an update on a multi-center experience [abstract]. Gastrointest Endosc 2010;71:AB229.

38. Rosch T, Daniel S, Scholz M, et al. Endoscopic treatment of chronic pancreatitis: a multicenter study of 1000 patients with long-term follow-up. Endoscopy 2002; 34:765.

39. Brand B, Kahl M, Sidhu S, et al. Prospective evaluation of morphology, function, and quality of life after extra-corporeal shockwave lithotripsy and endoscopic treatment of chronic calcific pancreatitis. Am J Gastroenterol 2000;95:3428.

40. Ammann RW, Muench R, Otto R, et al. Evolution and regression of pancreatic calcification in chronic pancreatitis. A prospective long-term study of 107 patients. Gastroenterology 1988;95:1018.

41. Sakorafas GH, Farnell MB, Farley DR, et al. Long-term results after surgery for chronic pancreatitis. Int J Pancreatol 2000;27:131.

42. Sherman S, Lehman GA, Hawes RH. Pancreatic ductal stones: frequency of successful endoscopic removal and improvement in symptoms. Gastrointest Endosc 1991;37:511.

43. Mariani A, Bernad JP, Provansal-Cheylan M, et al. Differences of pancreatic stone morphology and content in patients with pancreatic lithiasis. Dig Dis Sci 1991;36: 1509.

44. Papachristou GI, Baron TH. Complications of therapeutic endoscopic retrograde cholangiopancreatography. Gut 2007;56:854.

45. Thomas M, Howell DA, Carr-Locke D, et al. Mechanical lithotripsy of pancreatic and biliary stones: complications and available treatment options collected from expert centers. Am J Gastroenterol 2007;102:1896.

46. ASGE Technology Committee. Technology status evaluation report. Biliary and pancreatic stone extraction devices. Gastrointest Endosc 2009;70:603.

47. Familiari P, Spada C, Costamagna G. Dilation of a severe pancreatic stricture by using a guide wire left in place for 24 hours. Gastrointest Endosc 2007;66:618.
48. Costamagna G, Bulajic M, Tringali A, et al. Multiple stenting of refractory pancreatic duct strictures in severe chronic pancreatitis: long-term results. Endoscopy 2006;38:254.
49. Eisendrath P, Deviere J. Expandable metal stents for benign pancreatic duct obstruction. Gastrointest Endosc Clin N Am 1999;9:547.
50. Park do H, Kim MH, Moon SH, et al. Feasibility and safety of placement of a newly designed, fully covered self-expandable metal stent for refractory benign pancreatic ductal strictures: a pilot study. Gastrointest Endosc 2008;68:1182.
51. Sauer B, Talreja J, Ellen K, et al. Temporary placement of a fully covered self-expandable metal stent in the pancreatic duct for management of symptomatic refractory chronic pancreatitis: preliminary data. Gastrointest Endosc 2008;68: 1173.
52. Moon SH, Kim MH, Park do H, et al. Modified fully covered self-expandable metal stents with antimigration features for benign pancreatic duct strictures in advanced chronic pancreatitis, with a focus on the safety profile and reducing migration. Gastrointest Endosc 2010;72:86.
53. Sauerbruch T, Holl J, Sackmann M, et al. Disintegration of a pancreatic duct stone with extracorporeal shock waves. N Engl J Med 1986;314:818.
54. Inui K, Yamaguchi T, Ohara H, et al. Treatment of pancreatic duct stones with extracorporeal shock wave lithotripsy: results of a multicenter survey. Pancreas 2005;30:26.
55. Tandan M, Reddy N. Extracorporeal shock wave lithotripsy for pancreatic and large common bile duct stones. World J Gastroenterol 2011;17:4365.
56. Delhaye M, Arvanitakis M, Verset G, et al. Treatment for painful calcified chronic pancreatitis: extracorporeal shock wave lithotripsy versus endoscopic treatment: a randomized controlled trial. Gastroenterol Hepatol 2004;2:1096.
57. Kozarek R, Brandabur J, Ball T, et al. Clinical outcomes in patients who undergo extracorporeal shock wave lithotripsy. Gastrointest Endosc 2002;56:496.
58. Costamagna G, Gabbrielli A, Mutignani M, et al. Extracorporeal shock wave lithotripsy of pancreatic duct stones in chronic pancreatitis: immediate and medium-term results. Gastrointest Endosc 1997;46:231.
59. Farnbacher M, Schoen C, Rabenstein T, et al. Pancreatic duct stones in chronic pancreatitis: criteria for treatment intensity and success. Gastrointest Endosc 2002;56:501.
60. Adamek H, Jakobs R, Buttmann A, et al. Long term follow up of patients with chronic pancreatitis and pancreatic stones treated with extracorporeal shock wave lithotripsy. Gut 1999;45:402.
61. Lawrence C, Siddiqi F, Hamilton J, et al. Chronic calcific pancreatitis: combination ERCP and extracorporeal shock wave lithotripsy for pancreatic duct stones. South Med J 2010;103:505.
62. Shah R, Attwell A, Raijman I, et al. Per oral pancreatoscopy with intraductal holmium laser lithotripsy for treatment of main pancreatic duct calculi: a multi-center U.S. experience [abstract]. Accepted Digestive Disease Week 2012;75(4):AB154.
63. Kozarek RA. Pancreatic stents can induce ductal changes consistent with chronic pancreatitis. Gastrointest Endosc 1990;36:93.
64. Siegel J, Veerappan A. Endoscopic management of pancreatic disorders, potential risks of pancreatic prostheses. Endoscopy 1991;23:177.
65. Rossos PG, Kortan P, Haber GB. Complications associated with pancreatic duct stenting. Gastrointest Endosc 1992;38:252.

66. Burdick JS, Geenen JE, Venu R, et al. Ductal morphological changes due to pancreatic stent therapy: a randomized controlled study. Am J Gastroenterol 1992;87:1281.

67. Smith MT, Sherman S, Ikenberry SO, et al. Alterations in pancreatic ductal morphology following polyethylene pancreatic stent therapy. Gastrointest Endosc 1996;44:268.

68. Sherman S, Hawes RH, Savides TJ, et al. Stent-induced pancreatic ductal and parenchymal changes: correlation of endoscopic ultrasound with ERCP. Gastrointest Endosc 1996;44:276.

69. Freeman ML. Mechanical lithotripsy of pancreatic duct stones. Gastrointest Endosc 1996;44:333.

70. Sauerbruch T, Holl J, Sackmann M, et al. Extracorporeal shockwave lithotripsy of pancreatic stones. Gut 1989;30:1406.

71. Cahen DL, Couma DJ, Nio Y, et al. Endoscopic vs. surgical drainage of the pancreatic duct in chronic pancreatitis. N Engl J Med 2007;356:676.

Endoscopic Retrograde Cholangioscopy and Advanced Biliary Imaging

Amrita Sethi, MD

KEYWORDS

- POCS • SOC • Cholangioscopy • Narrow band imaging
- Confocal endomicroscopy • Intraductal ultrasound • Optical coherence tomography

KEY POINTS

- Advanced biliary imaging with catheter and probe-based instruments provide us with multiple modalities to enhance evaluation of biliary pathology.
- Fiber optic imaging allows for basic cholangioscopic imaging and characterization of mucosa. More advanced cholangioscopies provide enhanced features, such as narrow band imaging. Although these modalities theoretically offer promise, further improvements need to made in defining the role of such imaging.
- Probe-based confocal endomicroscopy offers possibilities of in vivo histologic imaging, and thus far validation studies suggest a promising diagnostic performance. Further study is needed, however, in interpreting imaging.
- Intraductal ultrasonography and optical coherence tomography offer promising diagnostic capabilities that rely on ductal wall patterns, which may be particularly beneficial when evaluating infiltrating lesions.
- It is unlikely that any one of these modalities will solve the dilemma of distinguishing malignancy in indeterminate strictures alone, but rather will need to be used in combination and in tandem with sampling techniques.

INTRODUCTION

Indeterminate biliary strictures remain an overwhelming challenge for the biliary endoscopist, and major advances have been made in biliary diagnostics. Over the past 10 to 15 years, biliary endoscopy has seen the emergence of multiple techniques that allow us to move beyond the interpretation of fluoroscopic images to the direct visualization of the bile duct. This visualization is in the form of white light; contrast-enhanced imaging, such as narrow band imaging (NBI); or in vivo histologic imaging with confocal endomicroscopy.

Division of Gastroenterology and Hepatology, Columbia University College of Physicians and Surgeons, 161 Fort Washington Avenue, Suite 862, Herbert Irving Pavilion, New York, NY 10032, USA
E-mail address: as3614@columbia.edu

Gastrointest Endoscopy Clin N Am 22 (2012) 451–460
doi:10.1016/j.giec.2012.05.008
1052-5157/12/$ – see front matter © 2012 Elsevier Inc. All rights reserved.

giendo.theclinics.com

The above-mentioned imaging modalities, available during endoscopic retrograde cholangioscopy (ERCP), are discussed in the article. In addition, their indications and current status of diagnostic performance are reviewed.

CHOLANGIOSCOPY

Cholangioscopy has been available for the past few decades, through the earlier advent of mother-daughter systems to the more recent, widely used peroral cholangioscopy (POCS) systems such as SpyGlass (Boston Scientific, Natick, MA, USA) to the less commercially available, charge-coupled device technology–based video cholangioscopes (Olympus, Center Valley, PA, USA). Significant work is also being done using upper endoscopes for direct POCS.

Using a catheter-type cholangioscope (Opticscope, Clinical Supply, Ltd, Tokyo, Japan), Fukuda and colleagues[1] described malignant strictures as having irregularly dilated and tortuous vessels (known as tumor vessels), ooze easily, and have irregular surfaces. Benign strictures were classified based on the presence of a smooth mucosa without neovascularization and papillogranular mucosa with no obvious mass. In addition, using these criteria during POCS increased the accuracy of diagnosing malignant strictures from 78.1% to 93.4% compared with ERCP with tissue sampling. The investigators did note that caution needed to be taken when visualizing inflammation because 5 of 38 patients received false positive cholangioscopic diagnoses. Kim and colleagues[2] reported that the presence of tumor vessels had a sensitivity of 61% in diagnosing malignancy, which increased to 96% when combined with biopsies. Tischendorf and colleagues[3] classified cholangioscopic findings in 12 patients with primary sclerosing cholangitis as suspicious for malignancy if there was an associated polypoid or villous mass, or an irregularly shaped ulceration. Using these criteria, cholangioscopy had a sensitivity of 92%, specificity of 93%, and negative predictive value of 97%. Benign strictures caused by scarring were described as smooth with no surface irregularities, whereas inflammatory strictures were described to have erythematous mucosa with erosive and ulcerous mucosa. Itoi and colleagues[4] described traditional white light cholangioscopy findings that were thought to represent normal mucosa, inflammation, scar, and cancer. Normal epithelium was described as having a flat surface (with or without pseudodiverticula) and a flat network of vessels compared with a bumpy surface with thin tortuous vessels that characterizes inflammation. Features suggestive of cancer included irregular papillary or granular lesions, and thin to thick tortuous vessels.[4]

Recently, long-term data have been reported describing single operator of cholangioscopy (SOC) using the SpyGlass system (Boston Scientific Natick, MA, USA) (**Figs. 1** and **2**). This cholangioscope is 3.4 mm in diameter, with a 1.2-mm accessory channel, and has a 2200-mm working length and can be passed through the working channel of standard duodenoscopes over a 0.035-mm guidewire. A 0.77-mm fiberoptic probe is passed through the 0.9-mm optic channel. Miniature biopsy forceps can be passed through the accessory channel. Irrigation can be provided through a 0.6-mm channel, which allows for improved visualization and clearance of debris.[5] In a large, multicenter prospective study, including 297 patients, 95 patients (47% with malignancy) were analyzed for the diagnostic performance of a SOC-based impression. SOC impression had a sensitivity of 78% (84% for intrinsic lesions vs 67% for extrinsic lesions), specificity of 82%, positive predictive value (PPV) of 80%, and negative predictive value (NPV) of 80%. Investigators thought that cholangioscopic findings changed management in 64% of patients. Criteria used to classify malignant and benign cholangioscopic diagnosis were not included in this study.[6] In a single center

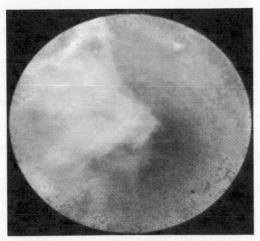

Fig. 1. Intraductal mass as seen during single operator cholangioscopy (SOC).

study using the same system, 36 patients with indeterminate strictures were evaluated with SOC. Malignancy was diagnosed by SOC impression in 21 of the 22 (95%) patients with a final diagnosis of malignancy. Three patients with benign strictures were incorrectly diagnosed with malignant strictures by SOC, and 79% were correctly classified as benign. The overall accuracy of differentiating malignant from benign disease based on SOC visual impression was 89% (sensitivity 95%, specificity 79%, PPV 88%, NPV 92%).[7]

CHOLANGIOSCOPY WITH VISUAL ENHANCEMENT

Contrast-enhanced endoscopy is widely used throughout the gastrointestinal (GI) tract to help delineate lesion margins, determine vascularization of lesions, and

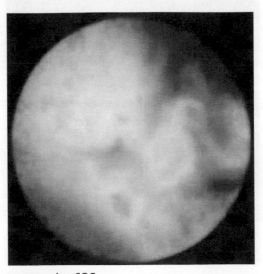

Fig. 2. Biliary stricture seen using SOC.

describe mucosal surface patterns. Enhanced image of the bile duct has been described with NBI, chromoendoscopy with methylene blue, and autofluorescence.

Chromocholangioscopy of the Bile Duct

Endoscopy using various dyes including crystal violet, indigo carmine, and methylene blue has been widely performed in the esophagus, stomach, and colon. Data regarding the use of methylene blue in the bile ducts suggest that it is feasible but may be limited by the presence of mucin, bile, and contrast.[8] Although mucosal patterns were enhanced, blood vessel delineation was unclear.[9] Thus, chromocholangioscopy seems to have a limited role based on the available literature.

NBI

The value of visualization with NBI over white light endoscopy in the GI lumen is well known. Two video cholangioscopes are currently available (CHF-B260 and CHF-BP260; Olympus Medical Systems, Tokyo, Japan) (**Figs. 3–5**), which can be used to provide NBI in the bile duct. Restricting light to 2 wavelengths, 415 nm and 540 nm, provides enhanced visualization of superficial mucosal capillary as well as pit patterns and thicker capillaries of the deeper tissues, respectively. Itoi and colleagues[4] demonstrated the feasibility of NBI in the bile duct using a video cholangioscope (CHF-B260; Olympus Medical Systems Tokyo, Japan) with an NBI system (CV-260SL processor, CVL-260SI light source; Olympus Tokyo, Japan) in determining lesion margins and identifying surface vessels. Twenty-one lesions in 12 patients were evaluated with NBI system and compared with those with conventional POCS. The investigators found that visualization of the surface structure and vessels with NBI was good or better than conventional imaging and excellent in a significantly greater number of lesions (57.4% vs 9.5%). Four lesions were detected by NBI that were not detected by white light endoscopy. Limitations to the use of NBI include the interference by the dark red appearance of blood and bile, as well as the lack of additional magnification systems on current cholangioscopes, a feature that is used to enhance NBI imaging of GI luminal epithelium.

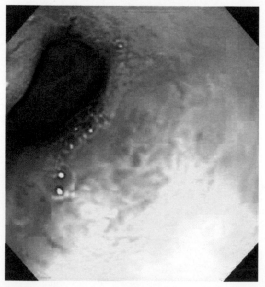

Fig. 3. Peroral cholangioscopy.

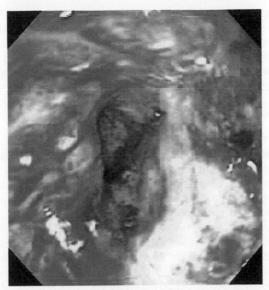

Fig. 4. Intraductal lesion seen using peroral cholangioscopy (Patient A).

Autofluorescence

Limited work has been performed to study the use of autofluorescence imaging (AFI) in the bile ducts. This technology first uses blue light as an excitation light after which autofluorescence is detected by using 2 hypersensitive cameras with red and green fields. In this imaging, normal mucosa is seen in green whereas neoplastic tissues change to dark green or black because of differences in the autofluorescence. Using the fiberoptic percutaneous transhepatic cholangioscope (PTCS) (FCN-15X; Pentax Co Ltd; and

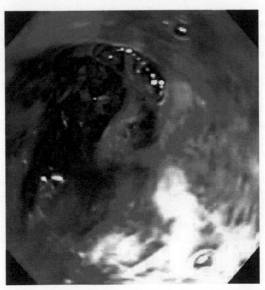

Fig. 5. NBI of Intraductal lesion seen using peroral cholangioscopy (Patient A).

CHF-P20; Olympus Medical Systems) or the fiberoptic POCS (FCP-9P, Pentax Co. Ltd Tokyo, Japan), Itoi and colleagues demonstrated that the addition of AFI could increase the diagnostic sensitivity of conventional PTCS from 88% to 100%; however, the specificity decreased from 87.5% to 52.5%.[10] The investigators concluded that future developments are needed to develop a more dedicated AFI video cholangioscopy system before it can be accurately used for enhanced biliary imaging.

CONFOCAL ENDOMICROSCOPY

The advent of confocal endomicroscopy has now allowed the biliary endoscopist to move from the radiographic interpretation of bile duct contours, to endoscopic epithelial imaging, to interpretation of the real-time histologic appearance of biliary epithelium. The principle of confocal microscopy is the focusing of light through a confocal aperture, which allows for elimination of scattered light above and below the plane. When scanned together in the same plane, each individual confocal point can provide dynamic images. This was first applied to visualize human intestinal tissue, ex vivo by Inoue and colleagues.[11] This confocal microscope system has been incorporated into 2 forms, a tip-based scope–based system, and a fiber-based confocal probe that is inserted through the conventional scopes. Only the probe-based confocal endomicroscopy (pCLE) system (Cellvizio; Mauna Kea Technologies, Paris, France) can be used to visualize biliary epithelium. A flexible biliary probe, called the CholangioFlex (Mauna Kea Technologies) can be passed either through a biliary catheter or the working channel of a cholangioscope. The probe has an external diameter of 0.94 mm, a field of view of 325 µm, a lateral resolution of 3.5 µm, with an optical thickness of 30 µm, and a 50 µm optical penetration. Intravenous fluorescein, which is absorbed by red blood cells, is given moments before the laser is activated and several subsurface features can be visualized. Early feasibility studies were performed to collect and identify features that would then be studied prospectively to validate a descriptive classification system of pCLE imaging (**Figs. 6** and **7**).[12,13] This classification system, known as the Miami classification, includes the following descriptive patterns: (1) dark or white bands, with or without branching, and with or without flow, either unidirectional or reversal of flow. These bands are classified as thin if up to 20 µm or thick if greater than 20 µm. (2) Dark clumps without epithelial features, (3) epithelial structures with or without the presence of glands, and (4) interstitial fluorescein leakage that appears as large areas of white surrounding other structures. Blinded consensus review of 112 sequences from

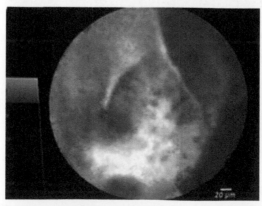

Fig. 6. Confocal endomicroscopy of an intraductal biliary lesion showing epithelium.

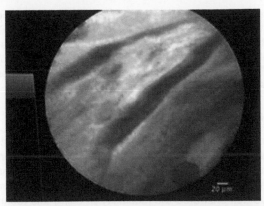

Fig. 7. Confocal endomicroscopy of an intraductal biliary lesion showing thick dark band.

47 patients with biliary strictures was performed. Sensitivity, specificity, PPV, and NPV of the findings of 2 or more of epithelial structures, thick bands greater than 40 mm (white or black), or dark clumps were 97%, 33%, 80%, and 80%, respectively. This was significantly improved when compared with standard tissue sampling, which had a sensitivity of 48%, specificity 100%, PPV 100%, and NPV 41%. Based on inter-observer variability assessed during this same study, the criteria were thought to be reproducible and there was moderate interobserver variability for most of the criteria. Thin dark bands had acceptable agreement as a marker of benign disease and visualization of epithelium had acceptable agreement in representing malignancy.[13,14]

Use of this technology is still developing and further study is currently being performed to further classify additional biliary findings. Futher study to determine the accuracy of confocal-based biliary diagnosis is needed to help define its role in advanced biliary diagnostic techniques.

INTRADUCTAL ULTRASONOGRAPHY

High-frequency (12–30 MHz) ultrasound probes that fit through the working channel of duodenoscopes can be used in the diagnosis of biliary malignancies and in distinguishing between intraductal masses, stones, and air bubbles that may appear as nonspecific filling defects on cholangiography. One probe has been designed to fit over a 0.035 guide-wire obviating sphincterotomy[15] and allowing selective cannulation of intrahepatic ducts. Both mechanical and electronic probes that, respectively, allow radial versus combined radial and linear scanning are available. Intraductal ultrasonography (IDUS) of the normal bile ducts demonstrates 2 to 3 sonographic layers, first a hypoechoic layer representing mucosa, muscularis propria, and fibrous layer of serosa. The second sonographic layer, a hyperechoic layer, represents subserosal adipose tissue, serosa, and the interface between serosa and adjacent organs. A variably seen third layer represents and interface echo.[16–19] Criteria used to diagnose malignancy include disruption of the normal echo layers, heterogeneity of the internal echo pattern, irregularity of the outer border, papillary surface, or a hypoechoic mass.[20–23]

IDUS has been demonstrated to have a high accuracy in diagnosing malignancy in indeterminate strictures when compared with other modalities or when added to baseline studies. Menzel and colleagues[21] demonstrated IDUS to have a higher accuracy compared with EUS (89% vs 76%, $P<.002$) in distinguishing benign versus malignant strictures in 56 patients. When evaluated in indeterminate strictures with negative cytology, Farrell and colleagues[24] demonstrated that IDUS added to ERCP had an accuracy of detecting malignancy of 92%, sensitivity of 90%, and specificity of 93%. Similarly, patients with malignant strictures tested positive with IDUS 2.06 times (95% CI, 1.37–3.10) that of ERCP in a study of 61 patients with painless jaundice and no mass on CT.[25] IDUS can accurately detect the proximal extent of biliary tumor in 92% of patients,[26] and has been shown to be more accurate when compared with cholangiography (84% vs 47%, P<.05).[20]

OPTICAL COHERENCE TOMOGRAPHY

The modality of optical coherence tomography (OCT) was introduced more than 20 years ago[27] and allows for high-resolution, cross-sectional, tomographic imaging of tissue by measuring the interference of low-power infrared light (750–1300 nm) reflected from the tissue and light reflected from reference mirrors. In vitro and in vivo studies have demonstrated the feasibility of using this technique to visualize multiple wall layers of the gut and pancreaticobiliary ducts, as well as visualize microscopic structures such as blood vessels, lymphoid aggregates, cyrpts, and glands.[28–32] In addition, neoplastic and non-neoplastic tissue could be differentiated.[33–35] The contrast of structures arises from the different optical reflectance properties of the tissue. OCT of the bile duct in humans was made possible by cannulating the duct with an OCT probe that was fit into a transparent biliary catheter and passed through the working channel of a standard ERCP scope.

Using 2 OCT criteria to diagnose malignancy, including unrecognizable layer architecture and the presence of large nonreflective areas compatible with tumor vessels, Arvanitakis and colleagues[36] evaluated the feasibility of OCT in detecting malignant biliary strictures in 35 patients. Using the midfocus OCT probe (Pentax Corporation, Tokyo, Japan/Lightlab Imaging Ltd, Boston, MA, USA; outer diameter 0.75 mm, depth of penetration 1 mm, resolution 10 μm) malignant strictures were diagnosed in 19 of the 25 (54%) patients compared with tissue as gold standard. The sensitivity of at least 1 or both OCT was 79% and 53%, respectively, and accuracy was 70% for both categories. When combining brushings/biopsies to at least 1 criteria, sensitivity increased to 84%.

SUMMARY

By allowing access to the bile duct, catheter and probe-based imaging tools can be used to provide multiple modalities of advanced imaging. Fiberoptic imaging allows for basic cholangioscopic imaging and characterization of mucosa. More advanced cholangioscopes allow for enhanced imaging with chromocholangioscopy narrow band functions, and autofluorescence. Although these modalities theoretically offer promise, further improvements need to be made in defining significance of findings. Probe-based confocal endomicroscopy offers exciting possibilities of in vivo histologic imaging, and thus far validation studies suggest a promising diagnostic performance. Further study is needed, however, in understanding and interpreting images. IDUS and OCT offer promising diagnostic capabilities that rely on ductal wall structure rather than mucosal and submucosal patterns, which may be particularly beneficial when dealing with infiltrating lesions. It is unlikely that any one of these modalities will solve the dilemma of distinguishing malignancy in indeterminate strictures, but rather will need to be used in combination and in tandem with sampling techniques.

REFERENCES

1. Fukuda Y, Tsuyuguchi T, Sakai Y, et al. Diagnostic utility of peroral cholangioscopy for various bile-duct lesions. Gastrointest Endosc 2005;62(3):374–82.

2. Kim HJ, Kim MH, Lee SK, et al. Tumor vessel: a valuable cholangioscopic clue of malignant biliary stricture. Gastrointest Endosc 2000;52(5):635–8.
3. Tischendorf JJ, Kruger M, Trautwein C, et al. Cholangioscopic characterization of dominant bile duct stenoses in patients with primary sclerosing cholangitis. Endoscopy 2006;38(7):665–9.
4. Itoi T, Neuhaus H, Chen YK. Diagnostic value of image-enhanced video cholangiopancreatoscopy. Gastrointest Endosc Clin N Am 2009;19:557–66.
5. Shah RJ, Adler DG, Conway JD, et al. Cholangiopancreatoscopy. Gastrointest Endosc 2008;68:411–21.
6. Chen YK, Parsi MA, Binmoeller KF, et al. Single-operator cholangioscopy in patients requiring evaluation of bile duct disease or therapy of biliary stones (with videos). Gastrointest Endosc 2011;74(4):805–14.
7. Ramchandani M, Reddy DN, Gupta R, et al. Role of single-operator peroral cholangioscopy in the diagnosis of indeterminate biliary lesions: a single-center, prospective study. Gastrointest Endoosc 2011;74(3):511–9.
8. Brauer BC, Fukami N, Chen YK. Direct cholangioscopy with narrow-band imaging, chromoendoscopy, and argon plasma coagulation of intraductal papillary mucinous neoplasm of the bile duct (with videos). Gastrointest Endosc 2008; 67(3):574–6.
9. Maetani I, Ogawa S, Sato M, et al. Lack of methylene blue staining in superficial epithelia as a possible marker for superficial lateral spread of bile duct cancer. Diagn Ther Endosc 1996;3(1):29–34.
10. Itoi T, Shinohara S, Takeda K, et al. Improvement of choledochoscopy-chromoendoscopy, autofluorescense imaging, or narrow-band imaging. Dig Endosc 2008; 67:574–6.
11. Inoue H, Igari T, Nishikage T, et al. A novel method of virtual histopathology using laser-scanning confocal microscopy in-vitro with untreated fresh specimens from the gastrointestinal mucosa. Endoscopy 2000;32:439–43.
12. Meining A, Frimberger E, Becker V, et al. Detection of cholangiocarcinoma in vivo using miniprobe-based confocal fluorescence microscopy. Clin Gastroenterol Hepatol 2008;6:1057–60.
13. Meining A, Shah RJ, Slivka A, et al. Classification of probe-based confocal laser endomicroscopy findings in pancreaticobiliary strictures. Endoscopy 2012;44: 251–7.
14. Meining A, Chen YK, Pleskow D, et al. Direct visualization of indeterminate pancreaticobiliary strictures with probe-based confocal laser endomicroscopy: a multicenter experience. Gastrointest Endosc 2011;74:961–8.
15. Ascher SM, Evans SR, Goldberg JA, et al. Intraoperative bile duct sonography during laparoscopic cholecystectomy: experience with a 12.5-MHz catheter-based US probe. Radiology 1992;185:493–6.
16. Kuroiwa M, Tsukamoto Y, Naitoh Y, et al. New technique using intraductal ultrasonography for the diagnosis of bile duct cancer. J Ultrasound Med 1994;13: 189–95.
17. Furukawa T, Naitoh Y, Tsukamoto Y, et al. New technique using intraductal ultrasonography for the diagnosis of diseases of the pancreatobiliary system. J Ultrasound Med 1992;11:607–12.
18. Fujita N, Yutaka N, Kobayahi G. Analysis of layer structure of the gallbladder all delineated by endoscopic ultrasound using the pinning method. Dig Endosc 1995;7:353–6.
19. Fujita N, Noda Y, Kobayashi G, et al. Staging of bile duct carcinoma by EUS and IDUS. Endoscopy 1998;30(Suppl 1):A132–4.

20. Kuroiwa M, Goto H, Hirooka Y, et al. Intraductal ultrasonography for the diagnosis of proximal invasion in extrahepatic bile duct cancer. J Gastroenterol Hepatol 1998;13:715–9.

21. Menzel J, Poremba C, Dietl KH, et al. Preoperative diagnosis of bile duct strictures–comparison of intraductal ultrasonography with conventional endosonography. Scand J Gastroenterol 2000;35:77–82.

22. Tamada K, Nagai H, Yasuda Y, et al. Transpapillary intraductal US prior to biliary drainage in the assessment of longitudinal spread of extrahepatic bile duct carcinoma. Gastrointest Endosc 2001;53:300–7.

23. Tamada K, Ueno N, Tomiyama T, et al. Characterization of biliary strictures using intraductal ultrasonography: comparison with percutaneous cholangioscopic biopsy. Gastrointest Endosc 1998;47:341–9.

24. Farrell RJ, Agarwal B, Brandwein SL, et al. Intraductal US is a useful adjunct to ERCP for distinguishing malignant from benign biliary strictures. Gastrointest Endosc 2002;56:681–7.

25. Stavropoulos S, Larghi A, Verna E, et al. Intraductal ultrasound for the evaluation of patients with biliary strictures and no abdominal mass on computed tomography. Endoscopy 2005;37:715–21.

26. Krishna NB, Saripalli S, Safdar R, et al. Intraductal US in evaluation of biliary strictures without a mass lesion on CT scan or magnetic resonance imaging: significance of focal wall thickening and extrinsic compression at the stricture site. Gastrointest Endosc 2007;66:90–6.

27. Huang D, Swanson EA, Lin CP, et al. Optical coherence tomography. Science 1991;254:1178–81.

28. Kobayashi K, Izatt JA, Kulkarni MD, et al. High-resolution cross-sectional imaging of the gastrointestinal tract using optical coherence tomography: preliminary results. Gastrointest Endosc 1998;47:515–23.

29. Cilesiz I, Fockens P, Kerindongo R, et al. Comparative optical coherence tomography imaging of human esophagus: how accurate is localization of the muscularis mucosae? Gastrointest Endosc 2002;56:852–7.

30. Testoni PA, Mariani A, Mangiavillano B, et al. Main pancreatic duct, common bile duct and sphincter of Oddi structure visualized by optical coherence tomography: an ex vivo study compared with histology. Dig Liver Dis 2006;38:409–14.

31. Tearney GJ, Brezinski ME, Bouma BE, et al. In vivo endoscopic optical biopsy with optical coherence tomography. Science 1997;276:2037–9.

32. Tearney GJ, Brezinski ME, Southern JF, et al. Optical biopsy in human gastrointestinal tissue using optical coherence tomography. Am J Gastroenterol 1997; 92:1800–4.

33. Testoni PA, Mangiavillano B, Albarello L, et al. Optical coherence tomography compared with histology of the main pancreatic duct structure in normal and pathological conditions: an 'ex vivo study'. Dig Liver Dis 2006;38:688–95.

34. Pitris C, Jesser C, Boppart SA, et al. Feasibility of optical coherence tomography for high-resolution imaging of human gastrointestinal tract malignancies. J Gastroenterol 2000;35:87–92.

35. Sergeev A, Gelikonov V, Gelikonov G, et al. In vivo endoscopic OCT imaging of precancer and cancer states of human mucosa. Opt Express 1997;1:432–40.

36. Arvanitakis M, Hookey L, Tessier G, et al. Intraductal optical coherence tomography during endoscopic retrograde cholangiopancreatography for investigation of biliary strictures. Endoscopy 2009;41:696–701.

Sampling at ERCP for Cyto- and Histopathologicical Examination

Jean-Marc Dumonceau, MD, PhD

KEYWORDS

- Endoscopic retrograde cholangio-pancreatography • Endoscopic ultrasonography
- Biliary stricture • Sampling • Cytology • Rapid on-site cytopathological examination

KEY POINTS

- Samples collected at the level of the biliopancreatic ducts allow for diagnosing malignancy with a specificity close to 100% but present a moderate sensitivity in most studies.
- A learning curve has been demonstrated for the team endoscopist-cytopathologist to reach a satisfactory sensitivity for the diagnosis of malignancy.
- Strategies to increase sensitivity for cancer diagnosis include the following:
  - Improved sampling method, using a grasping basket for cytopathological examination or combining brushing with biopsy sampling;
  - On-site microscopic examination of samples collected for cytopathological as well as histopathological examination;
  - The use of liquid-based cytology methods, combined or not with direct smears;
  - The use of ancillary diagnostic techniques to analyze cytopathological samples.

INDICATIONS

Sampling at endoscopic retrograde cholangio-pancreatography (ERCP) may be performed at the level of the duodenal papilla, of the biliary tree (including the right and left intrahepatic ducts), of the Wirsung duct and of the Santorini duct. In all of these locations except the papilla, sampling for cytopathological as well as histopathological examinations may be valuable.

- Papillary biopsy specimens may help in diagnosing autoimmune pancreatitis, immunoglobulin (Ig)G4-related sclerosing cholangitis, and ampullary neoplasm.[1]
- In the biliary tree, sampling is recommended every time that a stricture with no established or evident diagnosis (eg, anastomotic stricture following liver transplantation) is demonstrated. Dominant strictures in primary sclerosing cholangitis (PSC) pose a particular challenge.

Conflict of interest: None.
Division of Gastroenterology and Hepatology, Geneva University Hospitals, Rue Gabrielle Perret Gentil 4, 1211 Geneva, Switzerland
E-mail address: jmdumonceau@hotmail.com

Gastrointest Endoscopy Clin N Am 22 (2012) 461–477
doi:10.1016/j.giec.2012.05.006
1052-5157/12/$ – see front matter

- In the main pancreatic duct, sampling is usually recommended in case of dilation of unknown etiology without stricture (suspicion of intraductal papillary mucinous neoplasm) or in case of stricture. In patients who undergo endoscopic drainage of the main pancreatic duct for painful chronic pancreatitis, stricture sampling is usually performed at the time of first stent insertion because of the increased risk of pancreatic cancer in these patients.[2]

SAMPLE PROCUREMENT AND PREPARATION
Sampling for Cytopathological Examination

Material
Brushes are the most commonly used devices to sample the biliopancreatic ducts; they provide material for cytopathological examination. Models with a double-lumen catheter should be preferred for an easy, over-the-wire, manipulation (**Fig. 1**). The flagella at the tip of some brush models is useful in angulated ducts but it may hinder brush movements inside the intrahepatic ducts. Single-lumen cytology brushes are rarely used nowadays; they should not be used over the wire because retrieving the brush through the whole length of the catheter (to replace it with a guide wire) causes a substantial loss of cellular material on the inner side of the catheter.

Another device, the grasping basket, has been designed for sampling the biliary tree only (**Figs. 2** and **3**). Compared with brushes, it provides more material for cytopathological examination.[3] It is available in some countries only.

The Soehendra stent retriever is sometimes used to pass very tight strictures; in some cases material adequate for cytopathological examination may be retrieved from the serrations of the retriever.[4] In the same vein, Devereaux and colleagues[5] have placed 155 plastic stents into a fixative after retrieval from the biliary and pancreatic ducts. Cellular debris collected from the stent by a cytotechnician in the cytopathology laboratory allowed for diagnosing cancer with a sensitivity and specificity of 11% and 100%, respectively.

Methods
Sampling of biliopancreatic strictures for cytopathological examination is simple but meticulous execution is crucial to obtain decent results.

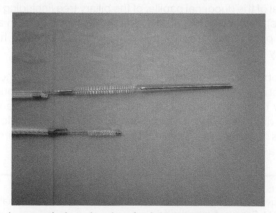

Fig. 1. Wire-guided cytopathology brushes for biliopancreatic sampling. Above, the Cytomax II brush whose flagella helps maintaining the brush inside the biliary lumen during back and forth movements in angulated ducts (Cook Endoscopy, Winston-Salem, NC, USA); below, the shorter RX cytology brush with no flagella (Boston Scientific, Natick, MA, USA).

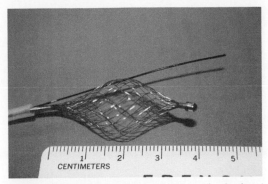

Fig. 2. Wire-guided grasping basket for biliary sampling. The basket is made of multiple stainless steel wires and measures approximately 15 mm in diameter (T E.I.M.E., Buenos Aires, Argentina). After deployment upstream from the stricture, the basket is withdrawn to grasp material from the biliary wall.

- First, all the material necessary for adequate sample preservation should be prepared before beginning the sampling procedure (**Fig. 4**). This is crucial because desiccation of monocellular layers obtained after smearing is extremely rapid.
- Standard brushing consists of introducing the brush/sheath as a unit over a guide wire through the stricture, withdrawing the unit brush/sheath immediately below

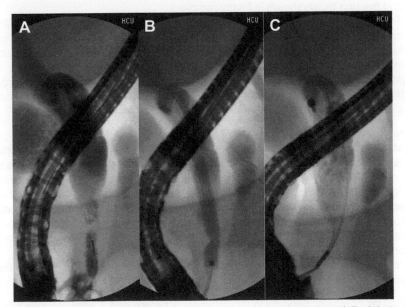

Fig. 3. Biliary sampling using a grasping basket (non–wire-guided model). (*A*) Contrast medium injection disclosed a dilation of the common bile duct upstream from an asymmetric stricture located at the tip of the sphincterotome. (*B*) After biliary sphincterotomy, the stricture was dilated using a 6-mm in-diameter balloon catheter (note the waist). (*C*) Full deployment of the grasping basket in the dilated portion of the duct, before withdrawal through the stricture.

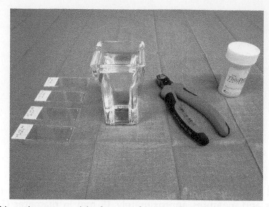

Fig. 4. Example of bench prepared *before* performing biliary brushing at ERCP. From left to right, glass slides labeled with patient identification; container filled with alcohol for preservation of smeared samples, wire cutters to separate the cytology brush from its supportive wire, and vial of PreservCyt solution (Cytic Corp., Boxborough, MA, USA). Bench preparation beforehand is critical to limit preservation artifacts.

the stricture, and then moving the brush back and forth precisely within the stricture at least 10 times. All these procedures should be performed under continuous fluoroscopic control with a sufficient magnification and amount of contrast medium in the biliary tree to ensure that the brush is correctly positioned within the stricture. Pulsed mode is recommended to limit radiation doses. The brush is then pulled into the sheath still located immediately below the structure and the unit brush/sheath is finally removed.

- If the grasping basket is used, the stricture is first dilated using a 6-mm balloon, then the basket (compressed in its sheath) is introduced upstream from the stricture, deployed and withdrawn through the stricture; the basket is finally retracted into its sheath still located immediately below the structure.
- After pancreatic brushing, a plastic pancreatic stent is usually inserted through the stricture to prevent post-ERCP pancreatitis, although the supporting evidence is weak in the absence of pancreatic sphincterotomy.[6,7]

Diagnostic accuracy

In 18 studies (**Table 1**), biliary brushing yielded a mean sensitivity for cancer diagnosis of 48%, with results extremely discordant between studies (from 9% to 93%); specificity was close to 100%. When averaging all studies listed in **Table 1**, biliary brushing was significantly less sensitive for the diagnosis of pancreatic as compared with biliary cancer (41% vs 59%, respectively; $P<.0001$). This lower sensitivity is generally attributed to the fact that biliary strictures caused by pancreatic cancer may be related to a compression, as opposed to an invasion, of the biliary wall and to a possible low cellularity and desmoplastic reaction in the case of pancreatic cancer.

Various methods have been tested to increase the sensitivity of sampling methods for cancer diagnosis at cytopathological examination:

- *Repeat brushing:* performing 2 brushings, 1 before and 1 after stricture dilation using 2 different brushes during a single ERCP, increased the sensitivity for cancer diagnosis in 2 studies (from 34% to 44% [$P = .001$] and from 40% to 45% [$P>.05$]).[8,9]
- *Rapid on-site cytopathological examination (ROSE):* if ROSE is unexpectedly negative for malignancy, some investigators repeat brushing.[10]

Table 1
Accuracy of biliary brushing to diagnose malignancy

First Author, Year	Overall	Sensitivity Pancreatic Cancer	Bile duct Cancer	Specificity
Venu et al,[58] 1990	77% (23/30)	60% (3/5)	80% (20/25)	100% (88/88)
Rupp et al,[59] 1990	93% (27/29)	91% (21/23)	100% (6/6)	88% (7/8)
Foutch et al,[60] 1991	45% (5/11)	0% (0/6)	100% (5/5)	100% (3/3)
Ryan,[61] 1991	34% (10/29)	30% (6/20)	44% (4/9)	100% (17/17)
Howell et al,[62] 1992	9% (2/22)	0% (0/18)	50% (2/4)	100% (5/5)
Kurzawinski et al,[63] 1993	64% (21/33)	65% (15/23)	60% (6/10)	100% (7/7)
Ferrari et al,[64] 1994	46% (18/39)	66% (16/29)	20% (2/10)	100% (22/22)
Ponchon et al,[25] 1995	33% (15/45)	15% (3/20)	44% (12/25)	97% (64/66)
Sugiyama et al,[27] 1996	48% (15/31)	36% (5/14)	59% (10/17)	100% (12/12)
Mansfield et al,[65] 1997	45% (20/44)	38% (10/28)	63% (10/16)	100% (2/2)
Vandervoort et al,[6] 1999	14% (8/56)	11% (5/46)	30% (3/10)	100% (37/37)
Glasbrenner et al,[66] 1999	53% (27/51)	35% (11/31)	80% (16/20)	90% (19/21)
Jailwala et al,[28] 2000	24% (18/76)	24% (11/46)	23% (7/30)	100% (29/29)
Farrell et al,[13] 2001	71% (20/28)	78% (14/18)	60% (6/10)	83% (10/12)
Fogel et al,[12] 2006	33% (42/126)	36% (32/88)	26% (10/38)	100% (8/8)
Kitajima et al,[23] 2007	67% (21/36)	60% (9/15)	71% (15/21)	100% (7/7)
Dumonceau et al,[11] 2008	43% (20/42)	38% (11/29)	69% (9/13)	100% (6/6)
Kawada et al,[10] 2011	84% (72/86)	71% (35/49)	100% (37/37)	100% (8/8)
Total	48% (387/814)	41% (207/508)	59% (180/306)	98% (351/358)

Data from Tamada K, Ushio J, Sugano K. Endoscopic diagnosis of extrahepatic bile duct carcinoma: advances and current limitations. World J Clin Oncol 2011;2:203–16.

- *Grasping basket:* in a randomized controlled trial (RCT) with blind examination of biliary samples collected using either a brush or the grasping basket, the grasping basket yielded a higher sensitivity for cancer diagnosis than brushing (80% vs 48%, respectively; $P = .018$).[11] Complications at 30 days were standard in terms of incidence (7%), severity, and type. In another study, the grasping basket was also found to yield more cellular material than brushing.[3] Another alternate sampling device, a long brush with stiff bristles, did not provide a higher sensitivity for cancer diagnosis compared with a standard brush despite a higher cellular yield.[12]
- *Stricture dilation:* stricture dilation aims at exposing deep tissue layers, which may be useful for example in case of biliary compression by a pancreatic cancer. Four studies were identified that compared the diagnostic yield of biliary brushing preceded or not by stricture dilation (**Table 2**).[8,9,11,13] No significant difference was found in terms of sensitivity for cancer diagnosis but a single study systematically used balloons (hence larger dilation) for stricture dilation so that this technique likely deserves further controlled trials.[11]

Biopsy Sampling

Material
Biopsy forceps of varying sizes and shapes may be used for sampling the biliary or pancreatic ducts under fluoroscopic control using a standard duodenoscope; forceps

Table 2
Influence of stricture dilation before biliary brushing

First Author, Year	Design for Stricture Dilation	Dilation Diameter, mm	Sensitivity for Cancer Diagnosis No Dilation	Dilation
Farrell et al,[13] 2001	Different patients, not randomized	3.3	85% (17/20)	57% (8/14)
de Bellis et al,[8] 2003	Brushing repeated in all patients following dilation	3.3–8.0	34% (40/116)	31% (36/116)
Ornellas et al,[9] 2006	Brushing repeated in all patients following dilation	3.3	40% (16/40)	28% (11/40)
Dumonceau et al,[11] 2008	Different patients, not randomized	6.0	35% (8/23)	59% (16/27)
Total			41% (81/199)	34% (71/207)

specifically designed for ERCP sampling are available (**Fig. 5**). If no sphincterotomy is performed, a biopsy forceps with a slide slit accepting a guide wire may be useful (available in some countries only).

Methods

The simplest technique consists of introducing a standard biopsy forceps transpapillary after endoscopic sphincterotomy. Because of the stiffness of standard biopsy forceps, sampling is facilitated by the insertion of a guide wire into the desired duct (for biliary sampling, the endoscope is positioned well below the papilla to lean the biopsy forceps against the duodenal wall). Biopsies are usually obtained from the inferior aspect of the stricture but they may also be obtained from the middle part of the stricture. Biopsy samples are placed into preservative as standard biopsies, except if ROSE is used (see later in this article). As pancreatic stenting for the prevention of post-ERCP pancreatitis is underused, it is important to recall that, in case of pancreatic sphincterotomy and biopsy sampling, the insertion of a plastic pancreatic stent is recommended.[7,14]

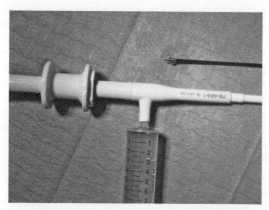

Fig. 5. Biopsy forceps specifically designed for biliary sampling. This biopsy forceps presents a single-side opening for tangential sampling, a malleable sleeve, and a port for contrast medium injection (Olympus, Tokyo, Japan).

Peroral cholangiopancreatoscopy is usually reserved for patients with an incomplete diagnosis after a workup using standard techniques because, compared with standard ERCP, it presents a series of limitations. These include a limited availability, more requirement for sphincterotomy, increased incidence of complications,[15] increased procedure duration and costs.[16] Furthermore, as far as sampling is considered, the effectiveness of peroral cholangiopancreatoscopy seems limited: in a prospective clinical cohort study that involved 15 endoscopy referral centers, sensitivity for cancer diagnosis using single-operator cholangioscopy-directed biopsy sampling was 49%.[17] The sensitivity calculated following the intention-to-diagnose principle is likely lower as procedural success of biopsy sampling was reported in approximately 90% of cases. Visual assessment of the bile duct wall may be more informative than sampling, in particular if ultrathin gastroscopes are used because they provide better images. This technique, named direct peroral cholangioscopy, allowed in a recent feasibility study for sampling some indeterminate biliary strictures; however, it is feasible in selected cases only and it still requires much improvement.[18]

Diagnostic accuracy

In 6 studies (**Table 3**), biopsy sampling at ERCP yielded a mean sensitivity for cancer diagnosis of 55%, with large variations between studies (from 32% to 82%); specificity was close to 100%. Contrary to a common belief, the diagnostic yield of biliary biopsy sampling is thus not much higher than that of biliary brushing (55% vs 48%, respectively; **Table 3** and **Table 1**). When averaging all studies listed in **Table 3**, biliary biopsy sampling was significantly less sensitive for the diagnosis of pancreatic as compared with biliary cancer (46% vs 63%, respectively; $P = .02$). This lower sensitivity is attributed to the frequent extraluminal location of pancreatic cancers.[19]

Various methods have been tested to increase the sensitivity of biopsy sampling for cancer diagnosis:

- *Number of biopsy samples, size of biopsy forceps:* in a RCT, 31 patients with a suspected hilar malignant biliary stricture were randomized to have 3 biopsies performed using either a standard or a jumbo biopsy forceps (7F or 9F, respectively); sampling was then repeated using the alternate biopsy forceps (3 biopsies again).[20] Overall, the sensitivity for cancer diagnosis based on 6 biopsies was 58.6% without a difference between standard and jumbo biopsies. The

Table 3
Accuracy of biliary biopsy sampling to diagnose malignancy

First Author, Year	Overall	Sensitivity Pancreatic Cancer	Bile Duct Cancer	Specificity
Kubota et al,[67] 1993	82% (18/22)	50% (2/4)	89% (16/18)	100% (5/5)
Ponchon et al,[25] 1995	45% (13/29)	46% (6/13)	44% (7/16)	97% (35/36)
Sugiyama et al,[27] 1996	81% (25/31)	71% (10/14)	88% (15/17)	100% (12/12)
Jailwala et al,[28] 2000	32% (24/76)	33% (15/46)	30% (9/30)	100% (10/10)
Tamada et al,[19] 2002	73% (27/37)	50% (6/12)	84% (21/25)	100% (18/18)
Kitajima et al,[23] 2007	58% (21/36)	60% (9/15)	57% (12/21)	100% (7/7)
Total	55% (128/231)	46% (48/104)	63% (80/127)	99% (87/88)

Data from Tamada K, Ushio J, Sugano K. Endoscopic diagnosis of extrahepatic bile duct carcinoma: advances and current limitations. World J Clin Oncol 2011;2:203–16.

sensitivity increased with the number of biopsies up to a maximum reached with 4 biopsies (37.9%, 48.3%, 55.2%, and 58.6% with 1, 2, 3, and 4 biopsies, respectively).

- *Site of biopsy sampling:* findings at percutaneous cholangiography in patients with a cholangiocarcinoma suggest that the number of biopsies required to reach a high sensitivity is related to the morphologic type of the tumor, with 3 biopsies from the tip of the lesion being sufficient with lesions of the papillary type, whereas more biopsies from the margins and within the stenosis would be required for lesions of the nodular or infiltrating type.[21]
- *ROSE:* biopsy samples may be examined on-site following a particular preparation (see later)[22]; biopsy sampling may thus be repeated until ROSE yields a result positive for malignancy.

Combined Techniques

Table 4 shows that combining brushing and biopsy sampling increases the sensitivity of biliary sampling for cancer diagnosis. The difference, in each particular study, between the less sensitive technique and the combination of both techniques ranged between 8% and 34%. This suggests that the increase in sensitivity is generally worth the hassle of combining both sampling procedures. Kitajima and colleagues have measured that the mean time required for brushing and for biopsy sampling was 2.4 and 8.5 minutes, respectively (this corresponded to 20% of the total procedure duration, and it is short compared with the additional time that would be required for endoscopic ultrasonography [EUS]-guided sampling).[23,24]

Of note, the yield of biopsy sampling was rarely reported following the intention-to-diagnose principle in the original studies. Therefore, the sensitivity of biopsy sampling may have been overestimated compared with that of brushing because biopsy sampling is less often successful than brushing. For example, Ponchon and colleagues[25] reported a sensitivity of biopsy sampling for cancer diagnosis of 43% (35 of 82 patients with a malignant diagnosis); this corresponds to a sensitivity of 26% in intention-to-diagnose because biopsy sampling was attempted in 134 patients with a malignant diagnosis. In the same study, brushing was successful in most attempted cases. Harewood and colleagues[26] reported successful biliary biopsy sampling in 39% of patients in whom biliary brushing had been obtained. On the other hand, Sugiyama and colleagues[27] reported successful biliary biopsy sampling and

Table 4
Sensitivity of brushing, biopsy sampling, and combined biliary sampling to diagnose malignancy

First Author, Year	n[a]	Brushing	Biopsy	Combination
Ponchon et al,[25] 1995	204	33%	26%	35%
Pugliese et al,[68] 1995	52	53%	53%	61%
Howell et al,[29] 1996	28	58%	31%	65%
Sugiyama et al,[27] 1996	43	48%	81%	81%
Jailwala et al,[28] 2000	133	26%	37%	48%
Kitajima et al,[23] 2007	60	72%	65%	74%
Weber et al,[69] 2008	58	41%	53%	60%

[a] Patients who had attempted biliary sampling with both methods were included; sensitivity was calculated following "intention-to-diagnose" principles if details sufficient for calculation were provided in the original articles.

brushing in 87% and 88% of 52 patients, respectively. In some studies,[28] the inclusion of patients with ampullary cancer also favored biopsy sampling in the comparisons listed in **Table 4**.

Three of the studies listed in **Table 4** used the Howell biliary introducer for at least one of the samplings (**Fig. 6**).[29] Because this device may be difficult to introduce into the desired duct due to its large diameter and rigidity,[23] some investigators use it mostly when the insertion of standard biopsy forceps is challenging.[22]

Bile Collection

Bile or pancreatic juice may be collected for cytopathological examination during ERCP (usually by aspiration upstream from a stricture) or via a nasobiliary or a nasopancreatic drain. A retrospective study compared the diagnostic yields of these techniques with other sampling methods in 214 patients who had a final diagnosis of malignancy.[30] The sensitivity for cancer diagnosis was 48% for brush cytology, 41% for biopsy forceps, 30% for aspirated bile cytology, and 24% for nasobiliary drain cytology (the latter figure dropped to 14% if the result of the first nasobiliary drain cytology only was taken into account, as bile sampling was repeated up to 4 times). In patients who had both brushing and biopsy samplings, bile collected through the nasobiliary drain yielded additional information in very few cases. Therefore, the investigators recommended this sampling technique only in patients with a suspected cholangiocarcinoma and neither brushing nor biopsy sampling at the time of ERCP. Nevertheless, bile is an important fluid for the discovery of new markers of biliopancreatic cancer.[31,32]

SAMPLE PROCESSING AND INTERPRETATION
Samples Collected for Cytopathological Examination

Smear preparation
Smears may be prepared using the conventional direct smear method or the liquid-based cytology (LBC) method.

- Direct smears are prepared in the endoscopy suite by rolling the brush onto a glass slide; this requires a certain level of skill and practice to avoid common pitfalls, including thick smears (cell details are obscured within clusters) and

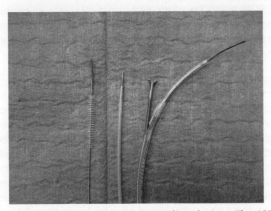

Fig. 6. Howell biliary introducer and dedicated sampling devices. The 10F introducer (*right*) presents a tapered tip and a lumen for a guide wire. The second lumen of the introducer measures 5F in diameter, exits at 4 cm from the tip of the catheter and accepts, from left to right, a brush, a 22-gauge needle, and a 5F biopsy forceps (Cook Endoscopy).

air-drying artifacts.[33] Smears may be allowed to dry or be fixed immediately using a spray or by immersion into 95% alcohol, depending on the cytopathologist's preference. Compared with the LBC method, direct smears present the advantage of permitting immediate naked-eye assessment of sample quality.

- Thin-layer LBC consists of making smears from cells suspended in a liquid medium using an automated machine. It eliminates the risk of air-drying/blood-clotting artifacts and decreases overlap of epithelial cells.[34] A part of the sample may also be used for cell-block preparation or stored for further additional preparation. Cell-block is a preparation in which the specimen is centrifuged into a pellet, formalin-fixed, paraffin-embedded, and sectioned for standard staining or ancillary tests, such as immunohistochemistry.

In 2 large nonrandomized studies that compared direct smears and LBC in a total of 1231 biliary and pancreatic specimens,[35,36] LBC allowed a significantly higher sensitivity for cancer diagnosis (60% vs 28% in one study and 53% vs 39% in the other) while maintaining a high specificity. The study that yielded the highest sensitivity indeed combined LBC and direct smears; this is usually achieved by making several direct smears and then placing the brush or the grasping basket into a vial containing a fixative or a transport medium. This combined method avoids discarding cellular material that sticks to the sampling device after smearing; it also allows for immediate assessment of sample quality on direct smears.

Bile or pancreatic juice is usually prepared for cytopathological examination by centrifugation at 1500 rpm for 5 minutes followed by preparation of a cytospin from the pellet, or cell-block preparation.[37,38]

Rapid on-site cytopathological examination

As it is performed for EUS-guided sampling in some centers (approximately 25% of European centers in a recent survey),[39,40] ROSE may also be used for ERCP samples. Kawada and colleagues[10] used ROSE to decide if brushing had to be repeated during ERCP; these investigators repeated brushing in 5 (7%) of the 76 patients for whom a cytopathological diagnosis of malignancy was obtained. In that study, the sensitivity for cancer diagnosis was one of the highest reported for biliary brushing (83%). Of note, performing biliary brushing twice (using 2 brushes) is known to significantly increase sensitivity for cancer diagnosis.[8]

ROSE during ERCP could be particularly cost-effective in centers where plastic biliary stents are not used in malignant strictures even if the tumor seems resectable.[41] In such settings, a self-expandable metal stent may be inserted during the first ERCP if a malignant stricture is diagnosed at ROSE.[42,43]

Delayed cytopathological examination

Cell characteristics that consistently indicate malignancy in the biliopancreatic tree have been described but they vary depending on the use of direct smears versus LBC.[34,44] Therefore, the role of a dedicated cytopathologist cannot be overstated. For example, Wight and colleagues[45] subjected 129 biliary brushings to re-reading by 2 dedicated pathologists without any clinical details. Compared with the initial diagnosis, more correct diagnoses were made by the 2 dedicated pathologists, with an increase in sensitivity for cancer diagnosis from 36% to 61% (specificity remained 100%). Even intraobserver agreement (ie, reproduction of the same diagnosis for the same sample by the same pathologist) may be lower than 80%.[46]

Use of clear categories in the cytopathological report is essential to ensure adequate patient management. The classical 5 diagnostic categories include normal, atypical considered reactive, highly atypical suspicious for cancer, malignant, and unsatisfactory. A broad diagnosis of "atypia" or "dysplasia" should not be used, as it is not clinically useful. A study showed that most of these "atypical" diagnoses could be reclassified in one of the classical diagnostic categories, increasing sensitivity for cancer diagnosis while maintaining 100% specificity.[44] Many groups of investigators have reported that using the category "highly atypical suspicious for cancer" as equivalent to malignant increases sensitivity for cancer diagnosis with no decrease in specificity.[47] However, this should be discussed and agreed on between the endoscopist and the cytopathologist based on local data because, using this approach, other groups of investigators have reported a relatively low specificity (83% in one large study).[48] In particular, interpretation of atypical diagnoses should be made with care in patients with PSC or with a stent in place before sampling for cytopathological examination.[6,13]

For all of these reasons, it may be extremely useful for endoscopists who do not work with a cytopathologist dedicated to biliopancreatic diseases to ask that ERCP cytopathology samples be sent to a cytopathologist with recognized experience in that field. The simplest way consists of sending glass slides by postal mail. Communication between the endoscopist and the cytopathologist is also essential to improve diagnostic accuracy; for example, if the cytopathologist provides feedback about sample quality, including cellular abundance and preservation. This is ideally achieved with ROSE.

In an attempt to increase sensitivity and interobserver agreement for the diagnosis of cancer, ancillary diagnostic techniques have been applied to ERCP samples. These include mutation analysis, digital image analysis, DNA ploidy analysis, methylation analysis, and fluorescence in situ hybridization.[49,50] These techniques are not widely available, however.

Samples Collected for Histopathological Examination

Biopsy specimens are usually placed into preservative and sent for standard histopathological processing and reading. Recently, ROSE has been adapted to ERCP biopsy specimens; this technique yielded a high sensitivity for cancer diagnosis (72% at ROSE and 76% at definitive pathologic examination) with 100% specificity in a series of 133 consecutive patients.[22] Briefly, biopsy specimens collected using a 5F or a 6F biopsy forceps were forcefully smashed between 2 dry glass slides to attempt creating a monolayer; they were immediately fixed, stained, and interpreted by an on-site cytopathologist. If the result was negative for cancer, the procedure was repeated a minimum of 10 times. The median number of biopsy specimens required for diagnosis was 3. Among patients with false-negative results, a true-positive result was obtained at ERCP sampling in an additional 4% of patients by fine-needle aspiration using the Howell biliary introducer or by histopathological examination of additional biopsies that had not been prepared for ROSE. EUS-guided sampling provided the diagnosis in an additional 10% of patients.

PARTICULAR DISEASES
IGG4-Related Sclerosing Cholangitis and Autoimmune Pancreatitis

IgG4-related sclerosing cholangitis may cause a biliary stricture; differentiation from PSC is clinically important. Pancreatography may provide a clue, as IgG4-related sclerosing cholangitis is frequently associated with autoimmune pancreatitis and an irregular narrowing of the main pancreatic duct. Treatment with corticosteroids is effective and a 2-week trial course of corticosteroids may be useful to confirm the diagnosis.

Biopsy sampling of the ampulla and of the common bile duct may help diagnosing IgG4-related sclerosing cholangitis by showing an increased number of IgG4-positive plasma cells at histopathological examination.[51,52]

Primary Sclerosing Cholangitis

Dominant strictures develop during the course of PSC in approximately half of patients.[53,54] Endoscopic treatment by balloon dilation is frequently performed in these patients because it improves survival without liver transplantation.[53,55] As PSC is a major risk factor for cholangiocarcinoma, the differential diagnosis of a dominant stricture versus a cholangiocarcinoma is of utmost importance. As no technique is sufficiently sensitive for cancer diagnosis, a combined approach of imaging techniques, serum markers, and biliary brushing plus biopsy sampling is recommended.[54]

A problem specific to cytopathological examination of biliary samples in PSC is the risk of false-positive diagnosis. A specificity of approximately 90% has been reported for biliary brushings collected in patients with PSC.[56] Harewood and colleagues[26] reported that most of their false-positive results at cytopathological examination occurred in patients with PSC. Of note, these false-positive results were observed during review of samples by cytopathologists who had no clinical information; the original sample examination by a pathologist who had clinical information did not yield a false-positive result. Therefore, it is important to inform the cytopathologist if a sample has been obtained in the setting of PSC.

HOW TO REACH A HIGH SENSITIVITY FOR CANCER DIAGNOSIS AT ERCP

A learning curve has been demonstrated for the diagnosis of cancer based on biliary brushing by the team endoscopist-cytopathologist: in a series of 406 biliary brushings, the sensitivity for cancer diagnosis increased from 44% in the initial third of cases to 71% in the final third of cases.[57] The problem is more important with cytopathologic as opposed to histopathologic examination, as shown by the much larger variations in sensitivity reported in **Table 1** versus **Table 3** (9%–93% vs 32%–82%, respectively). The problem of low sensitivity with ERCP samples, in particular brushing, is likely more important in the community because most published reports originate from specialized centers.

Logrono and colleagues[47] retrospectively reviewed the causes of false-negative results for 36 biliopancreatic brushing specimens. They identified 3 causes of errors that accounted for 76%, 14%, and 10% of false-negative results, respectively: sampling errors, air-drying artifacts, and interpretative errors at smear reading. These proportions will vary from one center to another, depending on the relative expertise in the team endoscopist-cytopathologist, but optimizing each of these steps is crucial to increase sensitivity for cancer diagnosis. Endoscopists with suboptimal results are likely to obtain rapid improvements by applying the following recommendations.

Sample Procurement and Preservation

Combine sampling for cytopathological and histopathological examinations.

Sampling for cytopathological examination:
- Prefer the grasping basket over brushes if available
- Use ROSE if available
- Prepare the material necessary for sample preparation and preservation before sampling

- Follow meticulously the sampling process described above; in particular for brushing, perform 10 passes precisely within the stricture under continuous fluoroscopic control (pulsed mode)
- If ROSE is unavailable, have a naked-eye check of direct smears (repeat sampling if material seems inadequate)
- Perform fixation of direct smears *immediately* (except if air-dried smears are preferred by the cytopathologist)
- Place the brush into liquid transport medium or preservative (request for LBC if this is not routinely performed)
- Provide at least the following information to the cytopathologist: (1) patient with a PSC or not and (2) presence of a stent before stricture sampling or not.

Sampling for histopathological examination:
- Use ROSE if available
- If ROSE is not available, obtain a minimum of 4 biopsies
- If biopsy sampling is difficult, consider stricture dilation with a 6-mm balloon or using the Howell biliary introducer.

Cytopathological Examination

- Send samples to a dedicated cytopathologist
- Ask for his or her feedback (eg, sample abundance and preservation)
- Ask for a diagnosis using 1 of 5 clear categories (the broad "atypical" or "dysplasia" categories should be banished)
- Consider a diagnosis of "highly atypical suspicious for cancer" as equivalent to cancer for clinical purposes if the cytopathologist agrees.

REFERENCES

1. Moon SH, Kim MH, Park DH, et al. IgG4 immunostaining of duodenal papillary biopsy specimens may be useful for supporting a diagnosis of autoimmune pancreatitis. Gastrointest Endosc 2011;71:960–6.
2. Lowenfels AB, Maisonneuve P, Cavallini G, et al. Pancreatitis and the risk of pancreatic cancer. International Pancreatitis Study Group. N Engl J Med 1993; 328:1433–7.
3. Dumonceau JM, Casco C, Landoni N, et al. A new method of biliary sampling for cytopathological examination during endoscopic retrograde cholangiography. Am J Gastroenterol 2007;102:550–7.
4. Brand B, Thonke F, Obytz S, et al. Stent retriever for dilation of pancreatic and bile duct strictures. Endoscopy 1999;31:142–5.
5. Devereaux BM, Fogel EL, Bucksot L, et al. Clinical utility of stent cytology for the diagnosis of pancreaticobiliary neoplasms. Am J Gastroenterol 2003;98: 1028–31.
6. Vandervoort J, Soetikno RM, Montes H, et al. Accuracy and complication rate of brush cytology from bile duct versus pancreatic duct. Gastrointest Endosc 1999; 49:322–7.
7. Dumonceau JM, Andriulli A, Devicro J, et al. European Society of Gastrointestinal Endoscopy (ESGE) Guideline: prophylaxis of post-ERCP pancreatitis. Endoscopy 2010;42:503–15.
8. de Bellis M, Fogel EL, Sherman S, et al. Influence of stricture dilation and repeat brushing on the cancer detection rate of brush cytology in the evaluation of malignant biliary obstruction. Gastrointest Endosc 2003;58:176–82.

9. Ornellas LC, Santos Gda C, Nakao FS, et al. Comparison between endoscopic brush cytology performed before and after biliary stricture dilation for cancer detection. Arq Gastroenterol 2006;43:20–3.

10. Kawada N, Uehara H, Katayama K, et al. Combined brush cytology and stent placement in a single session for presumed malignant biliary stricture. J Gastroenterol Hepatol 2011;26:1247–51.

11. Dumonceau JM, Macias Gomez C, Casco C, et al. Grasp or brush for biliary sampling at endoscopic retrograde cholangiography? A blinded randomized controlled trial. Am J Gastroenterol 2008;103:333–40.

12. Fogel EL, deBellis M, McHenry L, et al. Effectiveness of a new long cytology brush in the evaluation of malignant biliary obstruction: a prospective study. Gastrointest Endosc 2006;63:71–7.

13. Farrell RJ, Jain AK, Brandwein SL, et al. The combination of stricture dilation, endoscopic needle aspiration, and biliary brushings significantly improves diagnostic yield from malignant bile duct strictures. Gastrointest Endosc 2001;54:587–94.

14. Dumonceau JM, Rigaux J, Kahaleh M, et al. Prophylaxis of post-ERCP pancreatitis: a practice survey. Gastrointest Endosc 2010;71:934–9.

15. Sethi A, Chen YK, Austin GL, et al. ERCP with cholangiopancreatoscopy may be associated with higher rates of complications than ERCP alone: a single-center experience. Gastrointest Endosc 2011;73:251–6.

16. Neuhaus H. New techniques for direct biliary visualization: do we need them and what can be achieved? Gastrointest Endosc 2011;74:317–20.

17. Chen YK, Parsi MA, Binmoeller KF, et al. Single-operator cholangioscopy in patients requiring evaluation of bile duct disease or therapy of biliary stones (with videos). Gastrointest Endosc 2011;74:805–14.

18. Pohl J, Ell C. Direct transnasal cholangioscopy with ultraslim endoscopes: a one-step intraductal balloon-guided approach. Gastrointest Endosc 2011;74:309–16.

19. Tamada K, Tomiyama T, Wada S, et al. Endoscopic transpapillary bile duct biopsy with the combination of intraductal ultrasonography in the diagnosis of biliary strictures. Gut 2002;50:326–31.

20. Mutignani M, Galasso D, Familiari P, et al. Comparison of standard and jumbo endobiliary biopsy for histological diagnosis of hilar biliary strictures: interim report of a prospective randomized trial. Gastrointest Endosc 2008;67:AB169.

21. Tamada K, Satoh Y, Tomiyama T, et al. Multiple bile duct biopsies using a sheath with a side port: usefulness of intraductal sonography. AJR Am J Roentgenol 2001;176:797–802.

22. Wright ER, Bakis G, Srinivasan R, et al. Intraprocedural tissue diagnosis during ERCP employing a new cytology preparation of forceps biopsy (Smash protocol). Am J Gastroenterol 2011;106:294–9.

23. Kitajima Y, Ohara H, Nakazawa T, et al. Usefulness of transpapillary bile duct brushing cytology and forceps biopsy for improved diagnosis in patients with biliary strictures. J Gastroenterol Hepatol 2007;22:1615–20.

24. Dumonceau JM, Polkowski M, Larghi A, et al. Indications, results, and clinical impact of endoscopic ultrasound (EUS)-guided sampling in gastroenterology: European Society of Gastrointestinal Endoscopy (ESGE) Clinical Guideline. Endoscopy 2011;43:897–912.

25. Ponchon T, Gagnon P, Berger F, et al. Value of endobiliary brush cytology and biopsies for the diagnosis of malignant bile duct stenosis: results of a prospective study. Gastrointest Endosc 1995;42:565–72.

26. Harewood GC, Baron TH, Stadheim LM, et al. Prospective, blinded assessment of factors influencing the accuracy of biliary cytology interpretation. Am J Gastroenterol 2004;99:1464–9.

27. Sugiyama M, Atomi Y, Wada N, et al. Endoscopic transpapillary bile duct biopsy without sphincterotomy for diagnosing biliary strictures: a prospective comparative study with bile and brush cytology. Am J Gastroenterol 1996;91:465–7.

28. Jailwala J, Fogel EL, Sherman S, et al. Triple-tissue sampling at ERCP in malignant biliary obstruction. Gastrointest Endosc 2000;51:383–90.

29. Howell DA, Parsons WG, Jones MA, et al. Complete tissue sampling of biliary strictures at ERCP using a new device. Gastrointest Endosc 1996;43:498–502.

30. Yagioka H, Hirano K, Isayama H, et al. Clinical significance of bile cytology via an endoscopic nasobiliary drainage tube for pathological diagnosis of malignant biliary strictures. J Hepatobiliary Pancreat Sci 2011;18:211–5.

31. Farina A, Dumonceau JM, Lescuyer P. Proteomic analysis of human bile and potential applications for cancer diagnosis. Expert Rev Proteomics 2009;6: 285–301.

32. Farina A, Dumonceau JM, Frossard JL, et al. Proteomic analysis of human bile from malignant biliary stenosis induced by pancreatic cancer. J Proteome Res 2009;8:159–69.

33. Kocjan G, Chandra A, Cross P, et al. BSCC Code of Practice–fine needle aspiration cytology. Cytopathology 2009;20:283–96.

34. Ylagan LR, Liu LH, Maluf HM. Endoscopic bile duct brushing of malignant pancreatic biliary strictures: retrospective study with comparison of conventional smear and ThinPrep techniques. Diagn Cytopathol 2003;28:196–204.

35. Sheehan MM, Fraser A, Ravindran R, et al. Bile duct brushings cytology—improving sensitivity of diagnosis using the ThinPrep technique: a review of 113 cases. Cytopathology 2007;18:225–33.

36. Volmar KE, Vollmer RT, Routbort MJ, et al. Pancreatic and bile duct brushing cytology in 1000 cases: review of findings and comparison of preparation methods. Cancer 2006;108:231–8.

37. Davidson B, Varsamidakis N, Dooley J, et al. Value of exfoliative cytology for investigating bile duct strictures. Gut 1992;33:1408–11.

38. Noda Y, Fujita N, Kobayashi G, et al. Prospective randomized controlled study comparing cell block method and conventional smear method for pancreatic juice cytology. Dig Endosc 2012;24:168–74.

39. Polkowski M, Larghi A, Weynand B, et al. Learning, techniques and complications of endoscopic ultrasound-guided sampling in gastroenterology: ESGE Technical Guideline. Endoscopy 2012;44:190–206.

40. Dumonceau JM, Koessler T, van Hooft JT, et al. Endoscopic ultrasonography-guided fine needle aspiration: relatively low sensitivity in the endosonographer population. World J Gastroenterol 2012;18:2357–63.

41. Kahaleh M, Brock A, Conaway MR, et al. Covered self-expandable metal stents in pancreatic malignancy regardless of resectability: a new concept validated by a decision analysis. Endoscopy 2007;39:319–24.

42. Dumonceau JM, Tringali A, Blero D, et al. Biliary stenting: indications, choice of stents and results. ESGE Clinical Guideline. Endoscopy 2012;44:277–98.

43. Dumonceau JM, Heresbach D, Devière J, et al. Biliary stents: models and methods for endoscopic stenting. Endoscopy 2011;43:617–26.

44. Okonkwo AM, De Frias DV, Gunn R, et al. Reclassification of "atypical" diagnoses in endoscopic retrograde cholangiopancreaticography-guided biliary brushings. Acta Cytol 2003;47:435–42.

45. Wight CO, Zaitoun AM, Boulton-Jones JR, et al. Improving diagnostic yield of biliary brushings cytology for pancreatic cancer and cholangiocarcinoma. Cytopathology 2004;15:87–92.

46. Adamsen S, Olsen M, Jendresen MB, et al. Endobiliary brush biopsy: intra- and interobserver variation in cytological evaluation of brushings from bile duct strictures. Scand J Gastroenterol 2006;41:597–603.

47. Logrono R, Kurtycz DF, Molina CP, et al. Analysis of false-negative diagnoses on endoscopic brush cytology of biliary and pancreatic duct strictures: the experience at 2 university hospitals. Arch Pathol Lab Med 2000;124:387–92.

48. Duggan MA, Brasher P, Medlicott SA. ERCP-directed brush cytology prepared by the Thinprep method: test performance and morphology of 149 cases. Cytopathology 2004;15:80–6.

49. Fritcher EG, Halling KC. Advanced cytologic approaches for the diagnosis of pancreatobiliary cancer. Curr Opin Gastroenterol 2010;26:259–64.

50. Genevay M, Dumonceau JM, Pepey B, et al. Fluorescence in situ hybridization as a tool to characterize genetic alterations in pancreatic adenocarcinoma. Pancreas 2010;39:543–4.

51. Kubota K, Kato S, Akiyama T, et al. Differentiating sclerosing cholangitis caused by autoimmune pancreatitis and primary sclerosing cholangitis according to endoscopic duodenal papillary features. Gastrointest Endosc 2008;68:1204–8.

52. Kawakami H, Zen Y, Kuwatani M, et al. IgG4-related sclerosing cholangitis and autoimmune pancreatitis: histological assessment of biopsies from Vater's ampulla and the bile duct. J Gastroenterol Hepatol 2010;25:1648–55.

53. Stiehl A, Rudolph G, Klöters-Plachky P, et al. Development of dominant bile duct stenoses in patients with primary sclerosing cholangitis treated with ursodeoxycholic acid: outcome after endoscopic treatment. J Hepatol 2002;36:151–6.

54. Gotthardt D, Stiehl A. Endoscopic retrograde cholangiopancreatography in diagnosis and treatment of primary sclerosing cholangitis. Clin Liver Dis 2010;14: 349–58.

55. Gluck M, Cantone NR, Brandabur JJ, et al. A twenty-year experience with endoscopic therapy for symptomatic primary sclerosing cholangitis. J Clin Gastroenterol 2008;42:1032–9.

56. Ponsioen CY, Vrouenraets SM, van Milligen de Wit AW, et al. Value of brush cytology for dominant strictures in primary sclerosing cholangitis. Endoscopy 1999;31:305–9.

57. Stewart CJ, Mills PR, Carter R, et al. Brush cytology in the assessment of pancreatico-biliary strictures: a review of 406 cases. J Clin Pathol 2001;54: 449–55.

58. Venu RP, Geenen JE, Kini M, et al. Endoscopic retrograde brush cytology. A new technique. Gastroenterology 1990;99:1475–9.

59. Rupp M, Hawthorne CM, Ehya H. Brushing cytology in biliary tract obstruction. Acta Cytol 1990;34:221–6.

60. Foutch PG, Kerr DM, Harlan JR, et al. A prospective, controlled analysis of endoscopic cytotechniques for diagnosis of malignant biliary strictures. Am J Gastroenterol 1991;86:577–80.

61. Ryan ME. Cytologic brushings of ductal lesions during ERCP. Gastrointest Endosc 1991;37:139–42.

62. Howell DA, Beveridge RP, Bosco J, et al. Endoscopic needle aspiration biopsy at ERCP in the diagnosis of biliary strictures. Gastrointest Endosc 1992;38:531–5.

63. Kurzawinski TR, Deery A, Dooley JS, et al. A prospective study of biliary cytology in 100 patients with bile duct strictures. Hepatology 1993;18:1399–403.

64. Ferrari Júnior AP, Lichtenstein DR, Slivka A, et al. Brush cytology during ERCP for the diagnosis of biliary and pancreatic malignancies. Gastrointest Endosc 1994; 40:140–5.
65. Mansfield JC, Griffin SM, Wadehra V, et al. A prospective evaluation of cytology from biliary strictures. Gut 1997;40:671–7.
66. Glasbrenner B, Ardan M, Boeck W, et al. Prospective evaluation of brush cytology of biliary strictures during endoscopic retrograde cholangiopancreatography. Endoscopy 1999;31:712–7.
67. Kubota Y, Takaoka M, Tani K, et al. Endoscopic transpapillary biopsy for diagnosis of patients with pancreaticobiliary ductal strictures. Am J Gastroenterol 1993;88:1700–4.
68. Pugliese V, Conio M, Nicolò G, et al. Endoscopic retrograde forceps biopsy and brush cytology of biliary strictures: a prospective study. Gastrointest Endosc 1995;42:520–6.
69. Weber A, von Weyhern C, Fend F, et al. Endoscopic transpapillary brush cytology and forceps biopsy in patients with hilar cholangiocarcinoma. World J Gastroenterol 2008;14:1097–101.

Endoscopic Retrograde Cholangiopancreatography for Distal Malignant Biliary Stricture

Hiroyuki Isayama, MD, PhD[a],*, Yousuke Nakai, MD, PhD[a],
Kazumichi Kawakubo, MD, PhD[a], Hirofumi Kogure, MD, PhD[a],
Tsuyoshi Hamada, MD[a], Osamu Togawa, MD, PhD[b],
Naoki Sasahira, MD, PhD[a], Kenji Hirano, MD, PhD[a],
Takeshi Tsujino, MD, PhD[a], Kazuhiko Koike, MD, PhD[a]

KEYWORDS

- Obstructive jaundice • Endoscopic procedure • Biliary stenting • Cholecystitis
- Pancreatitis • Migration • Axial force • Metal stent

KEY POINTS

- Preoperative biliary drainage for pancreatic cancer may not be needed, but it may be useful with covered self-expandable metallic stents (SEMS) in neoadjuvant cases.
- Covered SEMS showed superior patency to uncovered SEMS, and may be the choice in unresectable distal obstruction.
- Each kind of SEMS has different mechanical properties and radial and axial force, which may influence the clinical results.
- Patients with tumor involvement of the orifice of the cystic duct were at high risk for post-SEMS cholecystitis.
- The risk factor of post-SEMS pancreatitis was nonpancreatic cancer, and using high axial force SEMS and sphincterotomy was not effective in preventing pancreatitis.
- Migration is one of the most important complications to be resolved. Lower axial force and providing an antimigration system may help prevent migration.
- Endoscopic ultrasonographic-guided biliary drainage is an effective salvage therapy, although it not well established. This procedure may avoid pancreatitis and cholecystitis.

INTRODUCTION

Endoscopic biliary stent placement is widely accepted as palliation for malignant biliary obstruction[1–4] or as a treatment of benign biliary stricture.[5,6] Many decades

---

Conflict of interest statement of corresponding author: No financial disclosure.
[a] Department of Gastroenterology, Graduate School of Medicine, The University of Tokyo, 7-3-1 Hongo, Bunkyo-ku, Tokyo 113-8655, Japan; [b] Department of Gastroenterology, Saitama Medical University International Medical Center, 1397-1 yamane Hidaka-shi 350-1298, Saitama, Japan
* Corresponding author.
E-mail address: isayama-tky@umin.ac.jp

have passed since self-expandable metallic stents (SEMS) were introduced, and although various biliary stent designs are now commercially available, no single ideal stent has yet been developed. An ideal stent should be patent until death, or surgery, in patients with resectable malignant biliary obstruction. Fewer complications, maneuverability, cost-effectiveness, and removability are also important factors. Alternatively, should we aim to develop a novel method for biliary drainage other than biliary stenting via endoscopic retrograde cholangiopancreatography (ERCP)? This article reviews the current status of biliary stenting for malignant biliary obstructions.

RESECTABLE MALIGNANT BILIARY OBSTRUCTION: PLASTIC, METAL, OR NO STENT?

Preoperative drainage is considered essential in patients with resectable periampullary malignancy, although biliary drainage itself can increase postsurgical complications[7,8] such as infection because of bacterial colonization or inflammation induced by preoperative drainage. Given the short time available, plastic stents (PS) are the standard method for preoperative drainage. Recently, van der Gaag and colleagues[9] conducted a randomized controlled trial (RCT) of preoperative biliary drainage in patients with obstructive jaundice caused by pancreatic cancer. Data suggested no benefit as a result of preoperative drainage in terms of complications or mortality. Overall serious complication rates were 39% and 74% ($P<.001$) and surgery-related complications were 37% and 47% in the early surgery and biliary drainage groups, respectively ($P = .14$). These investigators concluded that routine preoperative drainage increases complication rates and is not recommended. However, 46% of the biliary drainage group experienced complications, which appeared too high, as pointed out in the editorial in this issue.[10] Thus, more trials using either PS or SEMS are needed to confirm these investigators' conclusion and to alter clinical practice. Because the incidence of complications with currently available covered SEMS (CMS) is high, the role of CMS in the preoperative setting is limited.[11]

Neoadjuvant chemotherapy or chemoradiation therapy is a recent issue in borderline resectable pancreatic cancer. Most borderline resectable pancreatic cancer arises in the head of the pancreas and involves or abuts the major vessels. Longer stent patency is needed because the preoperative period in patients receiving neoadjuvant therapy is longer, and stent occlusion or stent-related complications cause cessation of neoadjuvant therapy. The occlusion rate of PS in patients with pancreatic cancer who underwent neoadjuvant chemoradiation therapy is as high as 55%.[12] Therefore, SEMS are an option for biliary drainage in this setting. Wasan and colleagues[13] compared SEMS and PS as preoperative biliary drainage in resectable pancreatic cancer. Although no stent-related postoperative complications occurred in either group, cholangitis or cholestasis was noted in 15% in the SEMS group and 93% in the PS group. In another retrospective study,[14] use of SEMS did not increase surgery-related complications (34%) or morbidity (0%); stent-related complication rates were 7% in SEMS and 45% in PS ($P<.0001$). These results suggest that SEMS offer longer stent patency without increasing complications and result in better cost-effectiveness in patients with resectable pancreatic cancer who require neoadjuvant treatment. However, these were retrospective studies at a single institution. Thus, the safety and efficacy, including cost-effectiveness,[15] of SEMS in patients with resectable pancreatic cancer should be confirmed in RCTs.[16–20]

UNRESECTABLE MALIGNANT DISTAL BILIARY OBSTRUCTION: COVERED OR UNCOVERED?

The ideal stent for unresectable malignant biliary obstruction should be easy to deploy, patent until death without complications, and provide antitumor effects.[21] The emergence of uncoated metal stents (UMS) prolonged stent patency significantly because of their larger diameter.[22–28] Historically, the cost-effectiveness of UMS has been debated. In patients with a poor prognosis (<3–6 months or liver metastasis),[29,30] PS are the reasonable choice in terms of cost-effectiveness. However, the prognosis of unresectable pancreatobiliary malignancy is improved by anticancer treatment, which necessitates longer stent patency.[31] As a result, a role for SEMS in unresectable distal malignant biliary obstruction is now frequently reported.[32–35]

The disadvantage of UMS is stent occlusion by tumor ingrowth or benign epithelial hyperplasia through the mesh. CMS were developed to overcome these disadvantages. The covering membrane of CMS, which does not allow embedding of the stent into the bile duct wall, prevents tumor ingrowth and epithelial hyperplasia. CMS were considered to be ideal when they first came into use,[36–48] but they have their own problems, which are discussed later.

So far, 5 RCTs[49–53] have been published, including 2 that used a percutaneous approach. We reported an RCT using diamond stents[49] and showed the superiority of hand-crafted polyurethane-covered diamond stents over uncovered diamond stents. In this study, tumor ingrowth was not observed in CMS and the stent occlusion rates were 14% and 38% in CMS and UMS, respectively. As a result, stent patency was significantly longer in CMS, but a trend toward higher complication rates of pancreatitis and cholecystitis was noted. Subsequently, 2 RCTs of a percutaneous approach confirmed a longer stent patency in pancreatic cancer[50] and extrahepatic bile duct cancer.[51] However, no significant differences were observed in 2 recently published RCTs.[52,53] CMS did not prevent tumor ingrowth in these studies, and stent migration was observed exclusively in 12%[52] and 3%[53] of patients.

Meta-analysis of these 5 RCTs[54] confirmed longer stent patency of CMS, but stent migration (relative risk, 8.11), tumor overgrowth (relative risk, 2.02), and sludge formation (relative risk, 2.89) were significantly higher with CMS. CMS were believed to increase cholecystitis or pancreatitis by blocking the orifice of the cystic duct or pancreatic duct with their covering membrane, but no significant increase in these complications was detected in this meta-analysis.

These studies clarified 2 points: what CMS can achieve and what problems CMS present. First, CMS can show significantly longer stent patency if the cover on CMS achieves its original goal of preventing tumor ingrowth. Second, the problems of stent migration or sludge formation should be resolved with CMS. Apparently, current commercially available CMS do not fulfill these requirements but we are still searching for an ideal one because the concept of CMS has been proved to be legitimate.

WHAT IS MISSING FROM THE COVERING MEMBRANE OF CURRENT CMS?

CMS were originally developed to prolong stent patency by preventing tumor ingrowth via the stent mesh. Therefore, the durability of the covering membrane is one of the most important factors of CMS. Various materials are used as the covering membrane, such as polyurethane, silicone, or expanded polytetrafluoroethylene (ePTFE). Hydrolysis from long-term bile exposure is the Achilles' heel of these covering materials. Durability comparing these materials was reported in a phantom model with bile flow[55,56] and silicone, which is used in commercially available covered Wallstents (Boston Scientific Corp., Natic, MA, USA) or covered WallFlex stents (Boston Scientific Corp., Natic, MA, USA), as being more resistant to hydrolysis than other materials.

Stent clogging from bacterial biofilm formation was extensively studied in PS. Medical treatment to prevent clogging was attempted using antibiotics or ursodeoxycholic acid, but these medications did not improve stent patency in clinical trials.[57]

CMS present similar problems because they are similar to an extremely large-pore PS. The covering membrane of ePTFE is prone to bacterial biofilm formation after bile exposure because of its rough and uneven surface.[56,58] Extensibility is another factor that can affect the mechanical characteristics, but no data are available about the influence of extensibility on different covering membranes.

The ideal covering membrane must be durable to long-term bile exposure and resistant to bacterial biofilms. More ex vivo data on this topic and their relation to clinical outcomes are awaited.

MECHANICAL PROPERTIES: ARE ALL SEMS THE SAME?

Mechanical properties of SEMS are defined by multiple factors such as stent design, type of wire, and covering materials. As a result of combinations of these variables, we proposed radial force (RF) and axial force (AF) as major mechanical properties that affect clinical outcomes.[59] RF is well known as an expanding force. AF is a straightening or recovery force when SEMS are bent, which is a new concept of stent properties. The measurement of RF and AF in various SEMS has been reported.[59]

RF affects stent patency in that dilation of biliary stricture and maintenance of luminal patency depend on the expanding force of SEMS. Two factors in RF exist in terms of time course. Immediate stent expansion at the time of stent deployment affects short-term outcomes, and chronic resistant force against tumor compression affects long-term outcomes. Insufficient expansion of SEMS immediately after deployment causes immediate stent occlusion by sludge or food impaction.[60] In general, the chronic resistant RF is higher than the immediate stent expanding force because SEMS are made of a type of shape-memory alloy. This characteristic means that SEMS sometimes expand partially immediately after deployment and then gradually expand to their full extent, even although the RF is high. To prevent immediate SEMS occlusion, balloon dilation after SEMS placement is effective in cases of partial expansion.

AF is considered to define conformability of SEMS in the bile duct and may have a greater relationship with clinical outcomes than RF. After deployment in the bile duct, SEMS are fixed at the stricture by the tumor and AF causes compression to the bile duct at both stent ends. As AF increases, so does the compression of the bile duct or cystic duct/pancreatic duct orifice. Clinically, this situation may cause kinking of the bile duct, cholecystitis, or pancreatitis. In addition, less conformability of SEMS in the bile duct leads to stent migration.

We have reported these correlations between mechanical properties and clinical outcomes. In general, AF affects clinical outcomes such as stent migration[43] and pancreatitis[61] more than RF. These results are useful in the development of new SEMS.

WHAT CAN WE DO TO PREVENT SEMS COMPLICATIONS?

Prevention of stent-related complications is important for the patient's quality of life and prolongation of survival. Stent-related complications necessitate reinterventions, impair the quality of life, and cause suspension of anticancer treatments. Stent migration, pancreatitis, and cholecystitis are problems with SEMS.

Stent migration is almost exclusively observed in CMS, although this characteristic provides removability. The removability of CMS expands their indications into the benign biliary stricture or bile leak.[62] It also makes reintervention easy at the time of stent dysfunction. CMS have also been considered to pose a risk factor of cholecystitis and pancreatitis, but recent studies including a meta-analysis[54] revealed no differences between CMS and UMS.

Several factors can cause stent migration: poor conformability of SEMS, lack of anchoring, tumor regression from chemotherapy, or stent excretion because of impacted sludge or food. The last cause should be considered as stent occlusion, but distinguishing between these 2 conditions clinically is difficult. Low AF and anchoring systems are the keys to preventing stent migration. We compared 2 CMS with different AFs (ComVi stent [Taewoong Medical, Seoul, Korea] and covered Wall-stent)[43] and the migration rate was significantly lower in the ComVi stent (2.1% vs 17.0%, respectively). The ComVi stent has a characteristic structure with a covering membrane sandwiched between 2 uncovered metallic stents, which achieves a low AF. Anchoring structures such as fins,[63] flares, and flaps[64] can also prevent stent migration. Park and colleagues[64] conducted a multicenter RCT of 2 CMS with flaps and flared ends in benign biliary stricture, and the anchoring flap was superior at preventing stent migration. Both stents were removable without complications. Recently, we conducted a multicenter prospective study of covered WallFlex stents.[65] Newly developed covered WallFlex stents are made of nitinol wires with low AF and have flared ends. As a result, stent migration rates were significantly lower in partially covered WallFlex stents (8%) than in partially covered Wallstents (17%). Stent removal was successful in 96%. Thus, we should develop CMS with effective anchoring systems and maintain removability.

Pancreatitis after SEMS placement is also an unsolved problem. Theoretically, compressing the orifice of the pancreatic duct causes pancreatitis. Cote and colleagues[66] reported a higher incidence of pancreatitis in SEMS compared with PS, but CMS or transpapillary stenting were not risk factors in a SEMS-specific analysis. Ternasky and colleagues[67] suggested deflection force on the pancreatic orifice by PS as a cause of postbiliary stent pancreatitis. Kawakubo and colleagues[61] conducted a multicenter retrospective study in the placement of 370 SEMS for malignant distal biliary obstruction, and the rate of pancreatitis was 6%. The rate of pancreatitis was 5.7% with CMS and 7.4% with UMS. The significant risk factors of pancreatitis were nonpancreatic cancer and SEMS with high AF. These results are in line with Ternasky and colleagues'[67] suggestion because high AF causes deflection and compression of the pancreatic duct. Thus, CMS do not increase the rate of pancreatitis but CMS with high AF are prone to both migration and pancreatitis.

Cholecystitis is another complication after SEMS placement,[68–70] which impairs the patient's quality of life. Previously, covering the orifice of the cystic duct was believed to cause cholecystitis after SEMS placement, but 2 retrospective studies[71,72] showed no significant differences in the rate of cholecystitis between UMS and CMS. These 2 studies both showed that tumor involvement at the orifice of the cystic duct is a significant risk factor for cholecystitis. We speculate that an expansion of SEMS causes the occlusion of the orifice of the cystic duct, which is narrowed and fixed by the tumor as opposed to patent and elastic in patients without tumor involvement. Intraductal ultrasonography (IDUS) is more accurate than cholangiography in the diagnosis of tumor involvement[73] and we routinely perform IDUS before SEMS placement to evaluate the risk of cholecystitis after SEMS placement. The risk factor for cholecystitis has been clarified but data are lacking on the prevention of cholecystitis after SEMS placement. Our preliminary analysis suggested that SEMS with high AF were more prone to cholecystitis. From our uni- and multivariate analysis of risk factors of cholecystitis, Tumor involvement of OCD (OR 5.34; 95% CI 2.19–13.0; $P = .0001$) and SEMS with high-AF (OR 5.18; 95% CI 1.69–22.6; $P = .027$) were significant risk factors (7% of cholecystitis among 356 cases placed at the OCD, presented at DDW 2012 by Isayama and colleagues).[74]

SEMS WITH ADDITIONAL FUNCTION

The attachment of the covering membrane to CMS provides the idea of using SEMS as local drug delivery platforms. The drug-eluting cardiac stents have already been in clinical use. In the cardiac stents, paclitaxel or sirolimus is used to prevent intimal hyperplasia. In biliary SEMS, paclitaxel-eluting stents were first reported in a porcine model.[75] The first human clinical trial[76] was reported in a case series of 21 patients. Stent occlusion was observed in 9 cases (sludge in 4, overgrowth in 3, and ingrowth in 2). Although the procedure itself was safe and feasible, its efficacy was unclear given the presence of tumor ingrowth in this study. Subsequently, a prospective RCT of paclitaxel-eluting CMS versus CMS[77] was conducted in 52 patients but no significant differences in stent patency or survival were detected. The study was underpowered and a larger study is needed to evaluate the efficacy of paclitaxel-eluting CMS. More recently, gemcitabine-eluting SEMS were reported in an animal study.[78] This stent seems promising because gemcitabine is the standard therapy in the treatment of advanced pancreatic or biliary tract cancer.

Other than a drug-eluting stent, brachytherapy via biliary stents[79] as anticancer treatment or holmium-166–incorporated covered stents in a porcine model[80] were also investigated. These stents can potentially work in preventing ingrowth as well as in anticancer treatments, resulting in both longer stent patency and better survival.

The other function to prolong stent patency can be seen in an antireflux stent. Dua and colleagues[81] conducted an RCT of PS with and without an antireflux valve. They reported longer stent patency with an antireflux valve (145 vs 101 days; $P = .002$). This study also confirmed the important role of duodenobiliary reflux as a cause of stent clogging. In a retrospective study on pancreatic cancer, we also reported that duodenal invasion was a risk factor of SEMS dysfunction.[82] Duodenal invasion causes congestion and increased pressure in the duodenum, which leads to more severe duodenobiliary reflux. Hu and colleagues[83] reported a feasibility of antireflux SEMS in 23 patients. Six stent malfunctions occurred as a result of tumor ingrowth ($n = 1$), tumor overgrowth ($n = 2$), and stent migration ($n = 3$). Occlusion by sludge or food impaction was not observed, and the median stent patency was as long as 14 months. Hu and colleagues presented the results of an RCT comparing this antireflux SEMS with conventional SEMS at Asian Pacific Digestive Week 2011, and showed the significantly longer stent patency in an antireflux stent than a conventional stent.

VARIOUS APPROACHES TO BETTER BILIARY DRAINAGE

One of the other approaches to keeping stent patency is local ablation of the tumor in the bile duct. Ablation of the tumor was reported using argon plasma coagulation or photodynamic therapy.[84–86] More recently, application of radiofrequency ablation (RFA) into the bile duct was reported.[87,88] RFA is now an established endoscopic treatment of Barrett esophagus.[89] In this study, a bipolar RFA probe that was 8Fr in diameter, 1.8 m long, and passed over a 0.89-mm (0.035-in) guidewire was used. The RFA probe was deployed successfully in 21 of 22 patients. The long-term results of stent patency or survival are still unknown, but given the high efficacy in Barrett esophagus, RFA in the biliary tract seems to be promising.

Problems with endoscopic biliary stent placement via ERCP arise because stents are transpapillary through the tumor. A novel approach of biliary drainage is endoscopic ultrasonographic-guided biliary drainage (EUS-BD), which creates a fistula between the gastrointestinal tract and biliary system without going through the tumor. EUS-BD was first reported as a salvage therapy in patients with failed ERCP or an inaccessible ampulla.[90–94] Hara and colleagues[95] reported on the safety and efficacy of EUS-BD in naive malignant biliary obstruction in a prospective study. The technical and functional success rates were 94% and 100%, respectively. This procedure may provide a paradigm shift to endoscopic treatments for malignant biliary obstruction if it can overcome the problems with SEMS placement via ERCP.

FUTURE PERSPECTIVE

Various SEMS are now commercially available and more and more stents are increasingly evaluated in clinical trials, but an ideal stent has not yet been found. The question is "Do we need a one-and-only ideal one-size-fits-all stent or should we focus on various tailor-made stents?" The indications of SEMS are expanding: benign biliary stricture or bile leak, preoperative drainage, or unresectable malignant biliary obstruction. In addition, prolonged survival as a result of chemotherapy has changed the role of biliary drainage in unresectable malignant biliary obstruction. Longer stent patency, fewer complications, and easier reinterventions are needed, but the importance of each factor varies according to the indications. Therefore, we should aim for tailor-made SEMS that are appropriate under various indications and conditions, although the concept of CMS to prolong stent patency is universal.

REFERENCES

1. Speer AG, Cotton PB, Russell RC, et al. Randomised trial of endoscopic versus percutaneous stent insertion in malignant obstructive jaundice. Lancet 1987;2: 57–62.
2. Shepherd HA, Royle G, Ross AP, et al. Endoscopic biliary endoprosthesis in the palliation of malignant obstruction of the distal common bile-duct–a randomized trial. Br J Surg 1988;75:1166–8.
3. Andersen JR, Sorensen SM, Kruse A, et al. Randomized trial of endoscopic endoprosthesis versus operative bypass in malignant obstructive jaundice. Gut 1989;30:1132–5.
4. Smith AC, Dowsett JF, Russell RC, et al. Randomised trial of endoscopic stenting versus surgical bypass in malignant low bileduct obstruction. Lancet 1994;344: 1655–60.
5. Barthet M, Bernard JP, Duval JL, et al. Biliary stenting in benign biliary stenosis complicating chronic calcifying pancreatitis. Endoscopy 1994;26:569–72.
6. Draganov P, Hoffman B, Marsh W, et al. Long-term outcome in patients with benign biliary strictures treated endoscopically with multiple stents. Gastrointest Endosc 2002;55:680–6.
7. Sohn TA, Yeo CJ, Cameron JL, et al. Do preoperative biliary stents increase post-pancreaticoduodenectomy complications? J Gastrointest Surg 2000;4:258–67 [discussion: 67–8].
8. Saleh MM, Norregaard P, Jorgensen HL, et al. Preoperative endoscopic stent placement before pancreaticoduodenectomy: a meta-analysis of the effect on morbidity and mortality. Gastrointest Endosc 2002;56:529–34.
9. van der Gaag NA, Rauws EA, van Eijck CH, et al. Preoperative biliary drainage for cancer of the head of the pancreas. N Engl J Med 2010;362:129–37.
10. Baron TH, Kozarek RA. Preoperative biliary stents in pancreatic cancer–proceed with caution. N Engl J Med 2010;362:170–2.
11. Tsujino T, Isayama H, Koike K. Preoperative drainage in pancreatic cancer. N Engl J Med 2010;362:1343–4 [author reply: 1346].
12. Boulay BR, Gardner TB, Gordon SR. Occlusion rate and complications of plastic biliary stent placement in patients undergoing neoadjuvant chemoradiotherapy

for pancreatic cancer with malignant biliary obstruction. J Clin Gastroenterol 2010;44:452–5.

13. Wasan SM, Ross WA, Staerkel GA, et al. Use of expandable metallic biliary stents in resectable pancreatic cancer. Am J Gastroenterol 2005;100: 2056–61.

14. Mullen JT, Lee JH, Gomez HF, et al. Pancreaticoduodenectomy after placement of endobiliary metal stents. J Gastrointest Surg 2005;9:1094–104 [discussion: 104–5].

15. Chen VK, Arguedas MR, Baron TH. Expandable metal biliary stents before pancreaticoduodenectomy for pancreatic cancer: a Monte-Carlo decision analysis. Clin Gastroenterol Hepatol 2005;3:1229–37.

16. Kahaleh M, Brock A, Conaway MR, et al. Covered self-expandable metal stents in pancreatic malignancy regardless of resectability: a new concept validated by a decision analysis. Endoscopy 2007;39:319–24.

17. Decker C, Christein JD, Phadnis MA, et al. Biliary metal stents are superior to plastic stents for preoperative biliary decompression in pancreatic cancer. Surg Endosc 2011;25(7):2364–7.

18. Pop GH, Richter JA, Sauer B, et al. Bridge to surgery using partially covered self-expandable metal stents (PCMS) in malignant biliary stricture: an acceptable paradigm? Surg Endosc 2011;25:613–8.

19. Singal AK, Ross WA, Guturu P, et al. Self-expanding metal stents for biliary drainage in patients with resectable pancreatic cancer: single-center experience with 79 cases. Dig Dis Sci 2011;56:3678–84.

20. Siddiqui AA, Mehendiratta V, Loren D, et al. Fully covered self-expandable metal stents are effective and safe to treat distal malignant biliary strictures, irrespective of surgical resectability status. J Clin Gastroenterol 2011;45: 824–7.

21. Isayama H, Nakai Y, Tsujino T, et al. Covered biliary metal stent: which are worse–the concepts, current models, or insertion methods? Gastrointest Endosc 2011; 73:1329–30 [author reply: 30–1].

22. Davids PH, Groen AK, Rauws EAJ, et al. Randomized trial of self-expanding metal stents versus polyethylene stents for distal malignant biliary obstruction. Lancet 1992;340:1488–92.

23. Knyrim K, Wagner HJ, Pausch J, et al. A prospective, randomized, controlled trial of metal stents for malignant obstruction of the common bile-duct. Endoscopy 1993;25:207–12.

24. Lammer J, Hausegger KA, Fluckiger F, et al. Common bile duct obstruction due to malignancy: treatment with plastic versus metal stents. Radiology 1996;201: 167–72.

25. Prat F, Chapat O, Ducot B, et al. A randomized trial of endoscopic drainage methods for inoperable malignant strictures of the common bile duct. Gastrointest Endosc 1998;47:1–7.

26. Kaassis M, Boyer J, Dumas R, et al. Plastic or metal stents for malignant stricture of the common bile duct? Results of a randomized prospective study. Gastrointest Endosc 2003;57:178–82.

27. Togawa O, Kawabe T, Isayama H, et al. Management of occluded uncovered metallic stents in patients with malignant distal biliary obstructions using covered metallic stents. J Clin Gastroenterol 2008;42:546–9.

28. Kogure H, Tsujino T, Yagioka H, et al. Self-expandable metallic stents for malignant biliary obstruction with an anomalous pancreaticobiliary junction. Surg Endosc 2008;22:787–91.

29. Yeoh KG, Zimmerman MJ, Cunningham JT, et al. Comparative costs of metal versus plastic biliary stent strategies for malignant obstructive jaundice by decision analysis. Gastrointest Endosc 1999;49:466–71.

30. Arguedas MR, Heudebert GH, Stinnett AA, et al. Biliary stents in malignant obstructive jaundice due to pancreatic carcinoma: a cost-effectiveness analysis. Am J Gastroenterol 2002;97:898–904.

31. Nakai Y, Isayama H, Kawabe T, et al. Efficacy and safety of metallic stents in patients with unresectable pancreatic cancer receiving gemcitabine. Pancreas 2008;37:405–10.

32. Lammer J, Klein GE, Kleinert R, et al. Obstructive jaundice: use of expandable metal endoprosthesis for biliary drainage. Work in progress. Radiology 1990; 177:789–92.

33. Irving JD, Adam A, Dick R, et al. Gianturco expandable metallic biliary stents: results of a European clinical trial. Radiology 1989;172:321–6.

34. Huibregtse K, Cheng J, Coene PP, et al. Endoscopic placement of expandable metal stents for biliary strictures–a preliminary report on experience with 33 patients. Endoscopy 1989;21:280–2.

35. Weston BR, Ross WA, Liu J, et al. Clinical outcomes of nitinol and stainless steel uncovered metal stents for malignant biliary strictures: is there a difference? Gastrointest Endosc 2010;72:1195–200.

36. Miyayama S, Matsui O, Terayama N, et al. Covered Gianturco stents for malignant biliary obstruction: preliminary clinical evaluation. J Vasc Interv Radiol 1997;8: 641–8.

37. Isayama H, Komatsu Y, Tsujino T, et al. Polyurethane-covered metal stent for management of distal malignant biliary obstruction. Gastrointest Endosc 2002; 55:366–70.

38. Kahaleh M, Tokar J, Conaway MR, et al. Efficacy and complications of covered Wallstents in malignant distal biliary obstruction. Gastrointest Endosc 2005;61: 528–33.

39. Nakai Y, Isayama H, Komatsu Y, et al. Efficacy and safety of the covered Wallstent in patients with distal malignant biliary obstruction. Gastrointest Endosc 2005;62: 742–8.

40. Soderlund C, Linder S. Covered metal versus plastic stents for malignant common bile duct stenosis: a prospective, randomized, controlled trial. Gastrointest Endosc 2006;63:986–95.

41. Park do H, Kim MH, Choi JS, et al. Covered versus uncovered wallstent for malignant extrahepatic biliary obstruction: a cohort comparative analysis. Clin Gastroenterol Hepatol 2006;4:790–6.

42. Yoon WJ, Lee JK, Lee KH, et al. A comparison of covered and uncovered Wallstents for the management of distal malignant biliary obstruction. Gastrointest Endosc 2006;63:996–1000.

43. Isayama H, Kawabe T, Nakai Y, et al. Management of distal malignant biliary obstruction with the ComVi stent, a new covered metallic stent. Surg Endosc 2009;24:131–7.

44. Ho H, Mahajan A, Gosain S, et al. Management of complications associated with partially covered biliary metal stents. Dig Dis Sci 2010;55: 516–22.

45. Isayama H, Yasuda I, Ryozawa S, et al. Results of a Japanese multicenter, randomized trial of endoscopic stenting for non-resectable pancreatic head cancer (JM-TEST)–covered Wallstent vs. double-layer stent. Dig Endosc 2011; 23:310–5.

46. Kawakubo K, Isayama H, Nakai Y, et al. Efficacy and safety of covered self-expandable metal stents for management of distal malignant biliary obstruction due to lymph node metastases. Surg Endosc 2011;25:3094–100.

47. Bakhru M, Ho HC, Gohil V, et al. Fully-covered, self-expandable metal stents (CSEMS) in malignant distal biliary strictures: mid-term evaluation. J Gastroenterol Hepatol 2011;26:1022–7.

48. Costamagna G, Tringali A, Reddy DN, et al. A new partially covered nitinol stent for palliative treatment of malignant bile duct obstruction: a multicenter single-arm prospective study. Endoscopy 2011;43:317–24.

49. Isayama H, Komatsu Y, Tsujino T, et al. A prospective randomised study of "covered" versus "uncovered" diamond stents for the management of distal malignant biliary obstruction. Gut 2004;53:729–34.

50. Krokidis M, Fanelli F, Orgera G, et al. Percutaneous palliation of pancreatic head cancer: randomized comparison of ePTFE/FEP-covered versus uncovered nitinol biliary stents. Cardiovasc Intervent Radiol 2011;34:352–61.

51. Krokidis M, Fanelli F, Orgera G, et al. Percutaneous treatment of malignant jaundice due to extrahepatic cholangiocarcinoma: covered Viabil stent versus uncovered Wallstents. Cardiovasc Intervent Radiol 2010;33:97–106.

52. Telford JJ, Carr-Locke DL, Baron TH, et al. A randomized trial comparing uncovered and partially covered self-expandable metal stents in the palliation of distal malignant biliary obstruction. Gastrointest Endosc 2010;72:907–14.

53. Kullman E, Frozanpor F, Soderlund C, et al. Covered versus uncovered self-expandable nitinol stents in the palliative treatment of malignant distal biliary obstruction: results from a randomized, multicenter study. Gastrointest Endosc 2010;72:915–23.

54. Saleem A, Leggett CL, Murad MH, et al. Meta-analysis of randomized trials comparing the patency of covered and uncovered self-expandable metal stents for palliation of distal malignant bile duct obstruction. Gastrointest Endosc 2011; 74:321–7, e1–3.

55. Kim DH, Kang SG, Choi JR, et al. Evaluation of the biodurability of polyurethane-covered stent using a flow phantom. Korean J Radiol 2001;2:75–9.

56. Bang BW, Jeong S, Lee DH, et al. The biodurability of covering materials for metallic stents in a bile flow phantom. Dig Dis Sci 2012;57(4):1056–63.

57. Galandi D, Schwarzer G, Bassler D, et al. Ursodeoxycholic acid and/or antibiotics for prevention of biliary stent occlusion. Cochrane Database Syst Rev 2002;3: CD003043.

58. Tsang TK, Pollack J, Chodash HB. Silicone-covered metal stents: an in vitro evaluation for biofilm formation and patency. Dig Dis Sci 1999;44:1780–5.

59. Isayama H, Nakai Y, Toyokawa Y, et al. Measurement of radial and axial forces of biliary self-expandable metallic stents. Gastrointest Endosc 2009;70:37–44.

60. Togawa O, Isayama H, Nakai Y, et al. Is the expansion rate of the covered metallic stents the predictive factor of patency? Gastrointest Endosc 2009;69:Ab144.

61. Kawakubo K, Isayama H, Nakai Y, et al. Risk factors for pancreatitis following transpapillary self-expandable metal stent placement. Surg Endosc 2012;26(3): 771–6.

62. Kahaleh M, Behm B, Clarke BW, et al. Temporary placement of covered self-expandable metal stents in benign biliary strictures: a new paradigm? (with video). Gastrointest Endosc 2008;67:446–54.

63. Hatzidakis A, Krokidis M, Kalbakis K, et al. ePTFE/FEP-covered metallic stents for palliation of malignant biliary disease: can tumor ingrowth be prevented? Cardiovasc Intervent Radiol 2007;30:950–8.

64. Park do H, Lee SS, Lee TH, et al. Anchoring flap versus flared end, fully covered self-expandable metal stents to prevent migration in patients with benign biliary strictures: a multicenter, prospective, comparative pilot study (with videos). Gastrointest Endosc 2011;73:64–70.
65. Isayama H, Mukai T, Itoi T, et al. The final Report of WATCH study; comparison of covered WAllflex StenT with covered Wallstent as historical control by Japanese Multicenter Study in cases with malignant distal biliary obstruction. Gastrointest Endosc 2011;73:AB188.
66. Cote GA, Kumar N, Ansstas M, et al. Risk of post-ERCP pancreatitis with placement of self-expandable metallic stents. Gastrointest Endosc 2010;72:748–54.
67. Tarnasky PR, Cunningham JT, Hawes RH, et al. Transpapillary stenting of proximal biliary strictures: does biliary sphincterotomy reduce the risk of postprocedure pancreatitis? Gastrointest Endosc 1997;45:46–51.
68. Gosain S, Bonatti H, Smith L, et al. Gallbladder stent placement for prevention of cholecystitis in patients receiving covered metal stent for malignant obstructive jaundice: a feasibility study. Dig Dis Sci 2009;55:2406–11.
69. Kawakubo K, Isayama H, Sasahira N, et al. Endoscopic transpapillary gallbladder drainage with replacement of a covered self-expandable metal stent. World J Gastrointest Endosc 2011;3:46–8.
70. Fumex F, Coumaros D, Napoleon B, et al. Similar performance but higher cholecystitis rate with covered biliary stents: results from a prospective multicenter evaluation. Endoscopy 2006;38:787–92.
71. Isayama H, Kawabe T, Nakai Y, et al. Cholecystitis after metallic stent placement in patients with malignant distal biliary obstruction. Clin Gastroenterol Hepatol 2006;4:1148–53.
72. Suk KT, Kim HS, Kim JW, et al. Risk factors for cholecystitis after metal stent placement in malignant biliary obstruction. Gastrointest Endosc 2006;64:522–9.
73. Nakai Y, Isayama H, Tsujino T, et al. Intraductal US in the assessment of tumor involvement to the orifice of the cystic duct by malignant biliary obstruction. Gastrointest Endosc 2008;68:78–83.
74. Isayama H, Kawakubo K, Nakai Y, et al. Self-expandable metallic stent with high axial force is the risk factor of cholecystitis. Gastrointestinal Endoscopy 2012;75 (4 Suppl):AB380.
75. Lee DK, Kim HS, Kim KS, et al. The effect on porcine bile duct of a metallic stent covered with a paclitaxel-incorporated membrane. Gastrointest Endosc 2005;61: 296–301.
76. Suk KT, Kim JW, Kim HS, et al. Human application of a metallic stent covered with a paclitaxel-incorporated membrane for malignant biliary obstruction: multicenter pilot study. Gastrointest Endosc 2007;66:798–803.
77. Song TJ, Lee SS, Yun SC, et al. Paclitaxel-eluting covered metal stents versus covered metal stents for distal malignant biliary obstruction: a prospective comparative pilot study. Gastrointest Endosc 2011;73:727–33.
78. Chung MJ, Kim H, Kim KS, et al. Safety evaluation of self-expanding metallic biliary stents eluting gemcitabine in a porcine model. J Gastroenterol Hepatol 2012;27(2):261–7.
79. Simmons DT, Baron TH, Petersen BT, et al. A novel endoscopic approach to brachytherapy in the management of Hilar cholangiocarcinoma. Am J Gastroenterol 2006;101:1792–6.
80. Won JH, Lee JD, Wang HJ, et al. Effects of a holmium-166 incorporated covered stent placement in normal canine common bile ducts. J Vasc Interv Radiol 2005; 16:705–11.

81. Dua KS, Reddy ND, Rao VG, et al. Impact of reducing duodenobiliary reflux on biliary stent patency: an in vitro evaluation and a prospective randomized clinical trial that used a biliary stent with an antireflux valve. Gastrointest Endosc 2007;65: 819–28.

82. Hamada T, Isayama H, Nakai Y, et al. Duodenal invasion is a risk factor for the early dysfunction of biliary metal stents in unresectable pancreatic cancer. Gastrointest Endosc 2011;74:548–55.

83. Hu B, Wang TT, Shi ZM, et al. A novel antireflux metal stent for the palliation of biliary malignancies: a pilot feasibility study (with video). Gastrointest Endosc 2011;73:143–8.

84. Harewood GC, Baron TH, Rumalla A, et al. Pilot study to assess patient outcomes following endoscopic application of photodynamic therapy for advanced cholangiocarcinoma. J Gastroenterol Hepatol 2005;20:415–20.

85. Kahaleh M, Mishra R, Shami VM, et al. Unresectable cholangiocarcinoma: comparison of survival in biliary stenting alone versus stenting with photodynamic therapy. Clin Gastroenterol Hepatol 2008;6:290–7.

86. Moon JH, Choi HJ, Ko BM. Therapeutic role of direct peroral cholangioscopy using an ultra-slim upper endoscope. J Hepatobiliary Pancreat Sci 2011;18: 350–6.

87. Itoi T, Isayama H, Sofuni A, et al. Evaluation of effects of a novel endoscopically applied radiofrequency ablation biliary catheter using an ex-vivo pig liver. J Hepatobiliary Pancreat Sci 2011. [Epub ahead of print].

88. Steel AW, Postgate AJ, Khorsandi S, et al. Endoscopically applied radiofrequency ablation appears to be safe in the treatment of malignant biliary obstruction. Gastrointest Endosc 2011;73:149–53.

89. Shaheen NJ, Sharma P, Overholt BF, et al. Radiofrequency ablation in Barrett's esophagus with dysplasia. N Engl J Med 2009;360:2277–88.

90. Giovannini M, Moutardier V, Pesenti C, et al. Endoscopic ultrasound-guided bilioduodenal anastomosis: a new technique for biliary drainage. Endoscopy 2001; 33:898–900.

91. Giovannini M, Dotti M, Bories E, et al. Hepaticogastrostomy by echo-endoscopy as a palliative treatment in a patient with metastatic biliary obstruction. Endoscopy 2003;35:1076–8.

92. Kahaleh M, Yoshida C, Kane L, et al. Interventional EUS cholangiography: a report of five cases. Gastrointest Endosc 2004;60:138–42.

93. Kahaleh M, Hernandez AJ, Tokar J, et al. Interventional EUS-guided cholangiography: evaluation of a technique in evolution. Gastrointest Endosc 2006;64:52–9.

94. Park do H, Jang JW, Lee SS, et al. EUS-guided biliary drainage with transluminal stenting after failed ERCP: predictors of adverse events and long-term results. Gastrointest Endosc 2011;74:1276–84.

95. Hara K, Yamao K, Niwa Y, et al. Prospective clinical study of EUS-guided choledochoduodenostomy for malignant lower biliary tract obstruction. Am J Gastroenterol 2011;106:1239–45.

Endoscopic Ultrasonography-Guided Endoscopic Retrograde Cholangiopancreatography

Endosonographic Cholangiopancreatography

Manuel Perez-Miranda, MD[a],*, Robert L. Barclay, MD, MSc, FRCP[b],
Michel Kahaleh, MD, AGAF[c]

KEYWORDS

- Endoscopic ultrasonography • Endoscopic retrograde cholangiopancreatography
- Cholangiopancreatography • Pancreatic access • Pancreatic drainage
- Biliary drainage

KEY POINTS

- Endoscopic retrograde cholangiopancreatography (ERCP) is the standard approach to gaining access to the biliary and pancreatic ductal systems, typically with therapeutic goals of stone extraction or decompression of an obstructed duct.
- In a small subset of cases anatomic constraints imposed by disease states or abnormal anatomy preclude ductal access via conventional ERCP.
- With the advent of endoscopic ultrasonography, with its unique capabilities of accurate imaging of the pancreas and biliary systems as well as ductal access via transmural puncture, there is now an alternative, endosonographic cholangiopancreatography (ESCP), to surgical and percutaneous radiologic approaches in situations inaccessible to ERCP.
- This article reviews the background, technical details, published experience and role of ESCP in clinical practice.

INTRODUCTION

Endoscopic retrograde cholangiopancreatography (ERCP) is the standard approach to gaining access to the biliary and pancreatic ductal systems, typically with therapeutic goals of stone extraction or decompression of an obstructed duct. However,

[a] Division of Gastroenterology and Hepatology, Hospital Universitario Rio Hortega, Valladolid University Medical School, Avenue Dulzaina, 2, 47012-Valladolid, Spain; [b] Rockford Gastroenterology Associates, University of Illinois College of Medicine at Rockford, 401 Roxbury Road, Rockford, IL 61107, USA; [c] Division of Gastroenterology and Hepatology, Department of Medicine, Weill Cornell Medical College, 1305 York Avenue, 4th Floor, New York, NY 10021, USA
* Corresponding author.
E-mail address: mperezmiranda@saludcastillayleon.es

Gastrointest Endoscopy Clin N Am 22 (2012) 491–509
doi:10.1016/j.giec.2012.05.004
1052-5157/12/$ – see front matter © 2012 Elsevier Inc. All rights reserved.

in a small subset of cases anatomic constraints imposed by disease states or abnormal anatomy preclude ductal access via conventional ERCP. Previously such situations prompted a percutaneous or surgical approach to therapy. However, with the advent of endoscopic ultrasonography (EUS), with its unique capabilities of accurate imaging of the pancreas and biliary systems as well as ductal access via transmural puncture, there is now an alternative to surgical and percutaneous radiologic approaches in situations inaccessible to ERCP: endosonographic cholangiopancreatography (ESCP). This article reviews the background, technical details, published experience, and role of ESCP in clinical practice.

BACKGROUND

ERCP is regarded as the standard, first-line method to achieve decompression of an obstructed biliary or pancreatic ductal system, with a technical success rate exceeding 90% and complication rate less than 10%.[1] However, surgically altered anatomy, variations of native anatomy, periampullary diverticula, and malignancy are circumstances that may preclude ERCP. In these situations, alternative means of biliary decompression include percutaneous transhepatic biliary drainage and surgical intervention. Percutaneous biliary drainage has a complication rate of 10% to 30%, with possible development of bile leak, bleeding, fistula formation, peritonitis, cholangitis, and stent occlusion; the death rate associated with percutaneous biliary drainage has been reported to be as high as 6%.[2] Although surgical biliary drainage is effective, it has been associated with a 2% to 5% rate of death and a 17% to 37% rate of morbidity.[3]

For highly experienced operators, reported success rates of pancreatic duct cannulation range from 90% to 98% for the major papilla and 90% to 95% for the minor papilla.[4] Several anatomic factors can be responsible for unsuccessful pancreatic duct cannulation at ERCP. For example, the papilla can be inaccessible because of either luminal obstruction of the upper gastrointestinal (GI) tract or surgically altered anatomy. Additional factors include inability to identify the pancreatic orifice of either the major or minor papilla, or benign or malignant strictures that impede deep cannulation of the pancreatic duct. Whereas a percutaneous approach in the setting of failed endoscopic biliary drainage is widely available and is associated with high success rates, an analogous percutaneous approach for pancreatic ductal access is neither as technically feasible nor as widely available. This shortcoming is due to multiple factors, including the deeper location of the pancreas compared with that of the intrahepatic bile ducts, smaller caliber ducts, and less compelling risk-benefit profiles of pancreatic ductal therapy.

Extensive experience with EUS-guided fine-needle aspiration (FNA) in and around the pancreas and extrahepatic bile duct provided the foundation for experimentation with EUS-guided biliary and pancreatic drainage. In contrast to a percutaneous approach, the proximity of these ducts to the gastroduodenal lumen, and therefore to the echoendoscope, is a distinct advantage of EUS-guided techniques. All experienced endosonographers are familiar with the close proximity of the common bile duct (CBD) and main pancreatic duct to the upper GI lumen. Indeed, in typical EUS-FNA cases, efforts are made to avoid these structures, which may lie near a targeted tumor mass.

Experience with EUS-guided biliary and pancreatic duct procedures has been expanding gradually since its inception, with the first description of EUS-guided cholangiopancreatography (ESCP) by Wiersema and colleagues[5] in 1996. Six variants of EUS-guided biliary and pancreatic duct drainage have been reported based on the ESCP paradigm (**Fig. 1**): ductal access under EUS coupled with ERCP-like

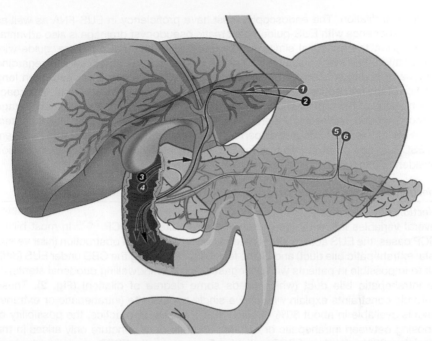

Fig. 1. The 3 potential ESCP access sites: intrahepatic (1, 2), extrahepatic (3, 4), and pancreatic (5, 6). After ductal access through any of them, drainage can be accomplished transmurally over an intraductal guide wire (1, 3, 6) via hepaticogastrostomy (1), choledochoduodenostomy (3), or pancreaticogastrostomy (6). Transpapillary guide-wire placement (2, 4, 5) allows both retrograde access via rendezvous ERCP and antegrade stent placement for biliary (2, 4) or pancreatic duct drainage (5). Rendezvous requires an accessible papilla and is preferable in benign disease. Antegrade transpapillary ESCP suits complex postoperative anatomy well, particularly when performed for palliation of malignant obstruction. Three access sites combined with 2 drainage routes gives rise to the 6 variant ESCP approaches. (*Reprinted from* Perez-Miranda M, de la Serna C, Diez-Redondo P, et al. Endosonography-guided cholangiopancreatography as a salvage drainage procedure for obstructed biliary and pancreatic ducts. World J Gastrointest Endosc 2010;2:214; with permission from Baishideng.)

instrumentation of the ducts under fluoroscopy. Just as ERCP gained wide acceptance because of its efficacy in clinical situations that previously necessitated more invasive approaches, in situations where ERCP is not possible, ESCP, another entirely endoscopic approach that obviates surgery or percutaneous intervention, has enormous potential and promise.

METHODS OF ESCP PROCEDURES
General Requirements and Patient Preparation

The procedure room and personnel requirements are the same as those for ERCP. Although ESCP is possible with small channel EUS scopes,[6] large-channel therapeutic echoendoscopes are preferable.[7,8] Similarly, EUS needles of a smaller caliber than 19-gauge represent an unnecessary burden, because the 0.018-in wires they allow are often associated with failed ESCPs, repeat 19-gauge punctures for larger wire passage, and the need for cautery access because of insufficient support for mechanical dilation. The endoscopist must have proficiency in EUS-FNA as well as ERCP. Experience with EUS-guided pancreatic pseudocyst drainage is also advantageous, given the technical similarities to ESCP in transmural puncture, guide-wire manipulation, and stent placement.[9] As with ERCP, there is no consensus regarding the type of sedation used for ESCP. However, given the complexity and often long duration of the procedure, standard conscious sedation may be insufficient. The coagulation status of the patient should be checked, and prophylactic antibiotic coverage is recommended. Increasingly, particularly in cases of anticipated difficulty at centers where ESCP has been adopted as part of the therapeutic algorithm, informed consent for ESCP is incorporated into that for ERCP, which obviates a separate discussion considering alternative drainage options.

Selection of Access Site and Drainage Route

Selection of access site
Several variables influence the choice of access site for ESCP.[7,8,10] In most biliary ESCP cases, the EUS access site is determined by the level of obstruction (hilar versus distal extrahepatic bile duct) and by the feasibility of imaging the CBD under EUS (difficult to impossible in patients with prior gastrectomy or indwelling duodenal stents) or the intrahepatic bile duct (which needs some degree of dilation) (**Fig. 2**). These anatomic constraints explain why only a single access site (intrahepatic or extrahepatic) is available in about 80% of biliary ESCP cases. In practice, the possibility of choosing between intrahepatic or extrahepatic bile-duct puncture only arises in the remaining 20% of biliary ESCP patients. For pancreatic ESCP cases, endosonographic access to the main pancreatic duct is typically obtained via transgastric puncture, although in cases where transduodenal access is feasible it is occasionally chosen by some investigators.[11]

Selection of drainage route
The choice between transpapillary and transmural drainage is influenced by the patient's anatomy and diagnosis (eg, CBD stone versus malignant stricture) and by operator preference. Patient-related factors cannot be altered in a given case other than by abandoning the procedure (ie, considering ESCP a failure if transpapillary guide-wire passage is unsuccessful and rendezvous is the only approach considered[12]) and opting for alternative therapies.[13] Technique and operator skill, however, can evolve and improve with practice. Whereas some investigators adhere to a single approach, such as rendezvous drainage only[12] or transduodenal access only,[14] those with broader experience in alternative approaches may be able to salvage a greater proportion of failed ERCPs by means of ESCP.[10,15,16]

ESCP Transpapillary Biliary Drainage (Rendezvous and Antegrade)

ESCP transpapillary biliary drainage entails gaining needle access to the intrahepatic or extrahepatic bile ducts under EUS guidance, followed by contrast injection (cholangiography), placement of a guide wire into the bile duct, then antegrade advancement of the guide wire across the native papilla (see **Fig. 1**). Subsequent biliary drainage is then effected either via a retrograde approach to the papilla (ie, ERCP) or EUS-guided rendezvous technique. Alternatively, drainage can be provided via an antegrade approach, typically following initial transgastric access into the intrahepatic system in patients with postoperative upper GI anatomy, for example, antegrade transgastric stent insertion[17] or balloon dilation[18] in patients with a strictured hepaticojejunostomy, or hilar lymph node recurrence causing obstructive jaundice after Roux-en-Y gastrectomy for gastric cancer (**Fig. 3**). For ESCP rendezvous, endoscopic access to the

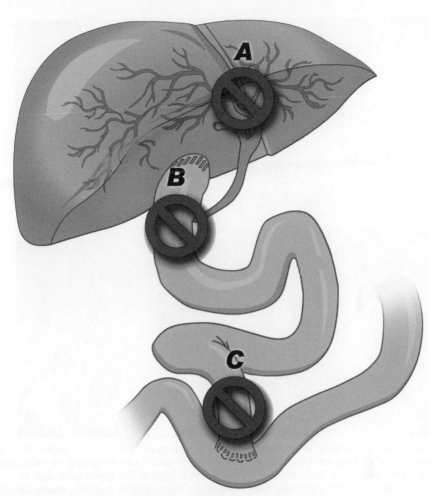

Fig. 2. Extrahepatic access is suitable for distal biliary obstruction in patients with native antroduodenal anatomy despite the presence of ascites or nondilated intrahepatic ducts (B). Any prior surgery involving distal gastrectomy with gastrojejunostomy (C) precludes EUS imaging of the CBD. Similarly, a hilar stricture with dilation of the left ductal system (A) requires intrahepatic access. Some of these patient specifics are present in 80% of carefully selected ESCP candidates, which limits the possibly overrated issue of operator's choice of approach to 20% of cases. (*Reprinted from* Perez-Miranda M, De la Serna C, Diez-Redondo P, et al. Endosonography-guided cholangiopancreatography as a salvage drainage procedure for obstructed biliary and pancreatic ducts. World J Gastrointest Endosc 2010;2:217; with permission from Baishideng.)

papilla is a prerequisite.[19,20] Usually this technique is prompted by obstruction or benign anatomic distortion of the native papilla, which precludes endoscopic retrograde biliary access. EUS-guided placement of a guide wire across the papilla then facilitates ERCP and conventional biliary therapy, for example, sphincterotomy and stone removal after failed cannulation caused by an intradiverticular papilla. For any kind of transpapillary drainage (antegrade or rendezvous) antegrade guide-wire passage from the puncture site into the small bowel is usually necessary, requiring

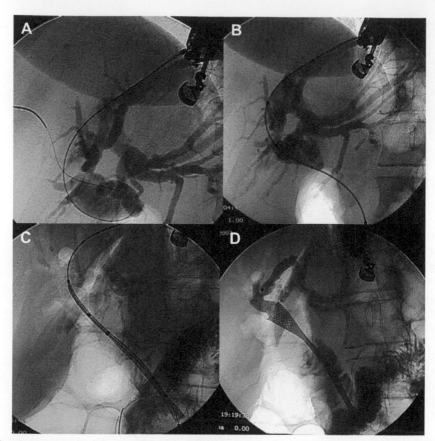

Fig. 3. Antegrade biliary stent insertion after intrahepatic EUS-guided access. Biliary obstruction after Roux-en-Y subtotal gastrectomy for gastric cancer caused by periportal lymph node recurrence. Note how after initial needle access the guide wire coils at the upper margin of the stricture and goes toward the right hepatic duct (*A*). Manipulation with a flexible catheter manages to redirect the guide wire downstream (*B*), allowing antegrade stent insertion (*C*) and deployment. Contrast injection after stent deployment demonstrates proper placement and function (*D*).

a nontransected duct. An exceptional case of successful rendezvous drainage of a transected bile duct has been reported.[21]

Guide-wire manipulation

The limiting step for transpapillary ESCP drainage is guide-wire manipulation.[13,15] The EUS needle does not allow the same free interplay over a guide wire as flexible ERCP catheters do, because the needle is rigid and has a sharp cutting edge. Repetitive or overly rapid to-and-fro movements of the needle over the wire risk shearing the guide wire or losing needle access to the duct.

Extrahepatic access for ESCP rendezvous EUS and fluoroscopy should be used to identify an access site as close to the papilla as possible, with a tangential needle orientation to the extrahepatic bile duct, before the actual puncture.[13,20,22] Postpuncture repositioning of the echoendoscope may be possible in cases with a largely dilated duct (eg, CBD above distal malignancy), although this carries the risk of losing needle access and possible procedural failure.

Intrahepatic access for rendezvous and antegrade ESCP Transpapillary guide-wire passage is usually more demanding from an intrahepatic (transgastric) than an extra-hepatic (transduodenal) access site.[13,23] After extrahepatic access, the guide wire can only pass either up or down the CBD. By contrast, after intrahepatic access it may pass peripherally to another left branch at every confluence, or to the right lobe ducts at the confluence of the right and left main hepatic ducts. Therefore, transpapillary guide-wire passage with intrahepatic ESCP often requires dilation of the puncture track to a degree similar to that required for transmural drainage, to allow intraductal passage of catheters or sphincterotomes.[24] These more maneuverable devices function to direct the guide wire toward the CBD and across the stricture and/or papilla. Traversing the papilla (or anastomosis) antegradely with a guide wire may require repeat needle puncture(s), reorientation, and different guide wires.[12] Despite all this instrumentation the process may end up in failure, particularly when antegrade guide-wire passage across the papilla is tried after pancreatic duct needle access (see later discussion).[25,26]

Scope exchange and retrograde guide-wire access for ESCP rendezvous
When guide-wire passage across the papilla is achieved, several loops of the wire should be advanced into the small bowel lumen to minimize the risk of dislodgment. For a rendezvous approach, the echoendoscope (with the needle attached) is removed carefully while the assistant feeds the wire into the needle at the same rate at which the endoscopist withdraws the scope-needle assembly.[19,20] The position of the guide wire is monitored fluoroscopically to prevent both looping in the stomach and dislodgment of the transpapillary looped wire from the small bowel (duodenum, or jejunum in patients with hepaticojejunostomy). After EUS scope removal, a duodeno-scope (or another scope of adequate length in patients with postoperative upper GI anatomy) is advanced alongside the guide wire while the assistant holds it under gentle traction from the patient's mouth to prevent looping.

Classic rendezvous Once the papilla is reached with a duodenoscope, the transpapil-lary guide wire can be grasped with a polypectomy snare or a rat-tooth forceps and retrieved upwards through the scope working channel, while the assistant feeds the guide wire from its proximal end into the patient's mouth in coordination. During the process of guide-wire retrieval up the scope working channel, considerable friction is encountered, which may result in guide-wire loss from the grasp of the snare or forceps. To avoid this friction and its attendant risk, some investigators take the alter-native step of removing the duodenoscope and the guide wire with a snare. Once the endoscope and guide wire exit from the patient's mouth, the endoscope is back-loaded over the wire down to the papilla.[13] Whatever the method of guide-wire retrieval up the working channel (with the endoscope inside or outside of the patient), standard ERCP devices can be threaded over the wire once it has exited from the endoscope channel. This technique is called classic rendezvous.

Parallel rendezvous Alternatively, once the duodenoscope reaches the papilla, a sphincterotome can be used for cannulation alongside the ESCP-placed wire (parallel rendezvous).[20,27] Although this approach saves the time-consuming and often cumbersome step of guide-wire retrieval through the duodenoscope, its disad-vantage is that it precludes dual traction (from the mouth end and from the endoscope end of the wire). For certain tight strictures (hilar bile duct or main pancreatic duct) that require stenting via ESCP, dual traction is a very useful ancillary technique that can obviate labor-intensive dilation before stenting.[8] Failed transpapillary stenting after fastidious ESCP rendezvous has been reported that may have been avoided via use of dual guide-wire traction.[28]

Non-rendezvous transpapillary ESCP drainage

Antegrade The hurdles of guide-wire manipulation with regard to antegrade transpapillary passage and retrograde retrieval have been detailed above, in particular the need to dilate the needle access tract to pass flexible devices that effectively redirect the guide wire antegradely across the stricture and the papilla in cases of intrahepatic access (see **Fig. 3**). Given the impossibility of imaging the CBD under EUS in patients with gastrectomy, intrahepatic access is the only one possible in most patients with postoperative upper GI anatomy. In these cases with long afferent limbs the papilla can be reached with enteroscopes, adding time and complexity to and already labor-intensive procedure. Antegrade stent insertion, or balloon dilation, over the transpapillary guide wire (as in percutaneous stent insertion) seem less cumbersome in this setting.[15,17,18]

Retrograde A simpler relatively overlooked approach to achieving retrograde transpapillary ductal access by ESCP has been described.[13,28,29] In some cases, either free-hand or standard wire-guided cannulation can be achieved despite prior unsuccessful ERCP, after the obstructed duct has been injected via ESCP with contrast medium or a mixture of contrast medium and methylene blue. Whether this approach is a "salvage" repeat ERCP after failed ESCP or a de novo ESCP-guided ERCP from the outset, the underlying premise is to enhance the visibility of an otherwise inconspicuous papilla or provide a guide for cannulation.

ESCP Transmural Biliary Drainage (EUS-Guided Choledochoduodenostomy and Hepaticogastrostomy)

As in endoscopic pseudocyst drainage, transmural duct drainage at ESCP is achieved by placing a stent across the GI wall and intervening structures into the target duct. For the bile duct there are 2 distinct sites that are typically chosen to place a transmural stent: (1) through the wall of the duodenal bulb into the CBD (EUS-guided choledochoduodenostomy [CDS]) or (2) below the cardia into the left hepatic duct (EUS-guided hepaticogastrostomy [HGS]). The terms CDS and HGS may not be literally accurate in certain cases, for example, after total gastrectomy and esophagojejunostomy whereby a transmural stent into the left hepatic duct is placed across the jejunal or distal esophageal wall, or when a transmural stent into the CBD enters the GI lumen through the wall of distal antrum rather than the duodenum.

EUS-guided choledochoduodenostomy

EUS-guided CDS involves stent placement across the duodenal wall into the extrahepatic bile duct. This procedure is considered in situations where conventional biliary cannulation and drainage is not possible, most often because of a tumor mass that either precludes luminal access to or obliterates the major papilla.

The linear-array echoendoscope is positioned in the long position, along the greater gastric curve, with the tip of the echoendoscope directed toward the hepatic hilum. This position allows endosonographic visualization of the dilated extrahepatic bile duct (**Fig. 4**). A 22-gauge or 19-gauge EUS-FNA needle is used to puncture the extrahepatic bile duct, under EUS guidance. After withdrawal of the stylet, bile is aspirated through the needle and a cholangiogram is obtained. Cholangiography is useful to confirm biliary access and to facilitate correct guide-wire placement. The guide wire

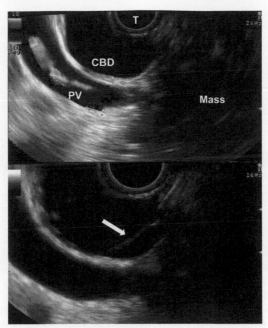

Fig. 4. EUS-guided extrahepatic duct access, US view. Transducer (T) in the duodenal bulb provides a longitudinal section of a dilated CBD above a pancreatic mass. Portal vein (PV) adjacent to the CBD is readily identified by color Doppler (*top*). A 0.035-in guide wire (*arrow*) through a 19-gauge EUS needle enters the CBD (*bottom*).

(preferably 0.025-in or 0.035-in, requiring a 19-gauge needle, or 0.018-in if using a 22-gauge needle) is advanced retrogradely into the intrahepatic biliary tree. Dilation of the transmural tract is then performed either with tapered biliary dilation catheters (6F, 7F, and 9F), needle knife, cystotome, or balloon dilation. Following tract dilation, a plastic or covered self-expandable metal stent is inserted through the choledochoduodenostomy over the guide wire, using similar techniques as for traditional ERCP stent placement.

EUS-guided hepaticogastrostomy
The proximity of the left lobe of the liver to the proximal stomach enables excellent EUS imaging of this portion of the liver. Experience with transgastric EUS-guided FNA of hepatic lesions demonstrated the utility and safety of needle puncture of the liver, with a low rate of complications. In patients with biliary obstruction, dilated intrahepatic biliary radicals may be well visualized via transgastric EUS.

The technique of EUS-guided HGS involves positioning of the linear-array echoendoscope tip against the proximal lesser gastric curve or cardia, where EUS can evaluate for dilated intrahepatic bile ducts. Color Doppler ultrasonography is used to distinguish bile ducts from blood vessels and to exclude intervening vessels in the needle path (**Fig. 5**). A dilated peripheral intrahepatic bile duct nearest to the EUS transducer is then punctured with a 22-gauge or 19-gauge EUS-FNA needle. After removal of the stylet, bile is aspirated and contrast dye is injected to obtain a cholangiogram. Bile aspiration and cholangiography are complementary means of confirming biliary access. Cholangiography is helpful to delineate ductal anatomy before guide-wire manipulation. If the step of aspirating bile is skipped, there is some risk

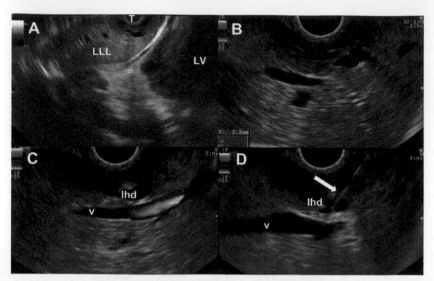

Fig. 5. EUS-guided left hepatic duct access, US view. (*A*) Transducer (T) below the cardia provides a longitudinal view of the caudad portion of the left ventricle (LV) and left liver lobe (LLL). (*B*) Close-up view allows identification of peripheral left hepatic duct (lhd) radicals of 3.3 mm. (*C*) Color Doppler readily identifies adjacent blood vessels (v). (*D*) Needle inside duct (*arrow*).

of parenchymal contrast injection when accessing small-diameter ducts, because the needle tip may mistakenly look intraductal on EUS while being located on a different plane. A guide wire (0.018-in if using a 22-gauge needle; 0.025-in or 0.035-in if using a 19-gauge needle) is advanced into the intrahepatic biliary tree. Next, steps are taken, as with CDS, to achieve transmural tract dilation and stent placement.

EUS-GUIDED PANCREATIC ACCESS AND DRAINAGE

The close proximity of the body and neck the pancreas to the posterior stomach enables excellent transgastric EUS imaging of the main pancreatic duct, the target for pancreatic ESCP. Extensive experience with EUS-guided FNA of pancreatic lesions has demonstrated a favorable safety profile of EUS-guided pancreatic needle puncture.

The technique of pancreatic ESCP involves positioning the linear-array echoendoscope tip against the posterior wall of the gastric body, where EUS can evaluate for a suitable site to access the main pancreatic duct. As with biliary ESCP, color Doppler ultrasonography is used to distinguish bile ducts from blood vessels and to exclude intervening vessels in the needle path. If the therapeutic goal is to gain access to the pancreatic duct for antegrade passage of a guide wire across the major or minor papilla, efforts are made to position the EUS scope tangentially, so that the direction of the needle puncture is toward the papilla, as this aids in subsequent threading of the guide wire into the pancreatic duct. Access to nondilated ducts is more challenging than to dilated ducts. The duct is punctured with a 22-gauge or 19-gauge EUS-FNA needle. Because motion from aortic pulsation and patient respiration often makes it challenging to maintain a secure position of the needle tip within the lumen of the pancreatic duct, particularly if the duct is of normal caliber, it is preferable to avoid use of the stylet and instead pass a guide wire as quickly as possible after gaining needle entry into the duct, with or without obtaining a prior pancreatogram. The EUS needle may be preloaded with contrast or a guide wire. The guide wire (0.018-in if using a 22-gauge needle; 0.025-in or 0.035-in if using a 19-gauge needle) is advanced deeply into the pancreatic duct, and across the papilla depending on the therapeutic context. If retrograde pancreatic therapy is required, the guide wire is left in place, with loops in the small bowel to anchor it. The echoendoscope and needle are withdrawn as a unit, taking careful precautions (see ESCP Rendezvous) to avoid wire displacement. In situations where the papilla is accessible, the duodenoscope is then passed to the papilla to perform the required therapy. If the goal is transmural drainage rather than transpapillary therapy, the EUS scope is left in place after gaining wire access to the pancreatic duct, and steps are taken (see Transmural Biliary Drainage) to achieve transmural tract dilation and stent placement.

In situations of failed retrograde pancreatography at ERCP where transpapillary therapy is desired, an ESCP approach using EUS-guided injection of contrast and methylene blue into the pancreatic duct, to guide retrograde pancreatic duct cannulation, has been used with a reasonable success rate,[29] obviating transgastric guide-wire placement in most cases of transpapillary pancreatic therapy. This approach is analogous to that described for biliary ESCP (see Transpapillary Biliary Drainage). Some investigators advocate parenteral octreotide administration after failed pancreatic duct access,[20,25] to minimize pancreatic secretion and prevent retroperitoneal leakage through the puncture track, although its efficacy has not been established.

CREATION OF TRANSMURAL FISTULOUS TRACT IN ESCP

The limiting step for transmural drainage is the creation of a fistulous track between the puncture site on the GI wall and the duct to allow stent placement. This approach requires at least bougie (stepped dilating catheters) or balloon dilation, and sometimes cautery with a needle knife or a fistulotome. Cautery may pose an increased risk for complications, although some investigators favor it for transduodenal access to the CBD when transmural drainage (CDS) is the final goal.[30] A needle knife (or fistulotome) is advanced either free-hand or wire-guided into the CBD. Prior fine-needle (22-gauge) ESCP cholangiography may or may not be performed to allow the added benefit of fluoroscopy during access to the CBD (because cautery creates EUS artifacts). For fistulotome access, ESCP is used routinely for prior intraductal wire placement. Because the driving mechanism for fistula formation is cautery (as opposed to mechanical, pushing force), a 0.018-in or 0.021-in guide wire is sufficient.[31] Given that 22-gauge needles can accommodate these thinner wires, cautery access obviates the use of stiff, larger 19-gauge needles. 19-Gauge needles may become cumbersome during transduodenal access because the echoendoscope is in a longer, looped position in comparison with intrahepatic access.

If one elects to create a fistulous tract using only mechanical dilation without cautery, it is important to maintain the endosonographic plane of view.[9,16,32] This is an important but underappreciated technical detail that has received little attention in previous reports of EUS-guided biliary drainage. The EUS plane may be easily lost if the operator shifts from sonographic monitoring of ductal access to endoscopic control once the guide wire is inside the duct, as one would do for transgastric pseudocyst drainage with the classic "blind" (ie, no EUS guidance) approach. In other words, to keep the appropriate sonographic plane and guide-wire axis of approach, the echoendoscope tip must remain in the same position throughout the steps of fistula-tract dilation and stent insertion as it was when the needle first punctured the duct. If one adheres carefully to this technique, only a minority of patients will fail mechanical track dilation and require additional cautery access with an over-the-wire device such as a needle knife or a fistulotome.[32] This concept requires the concerted, counterintuitive focus of the operator, as there is a deep-seated therapeutic endoscopist impulse to keep in endoscopic view a guide wire over which a device or stent is being advanced. In the setting of fistula creation via ESCP, this impulse should be deliberately ignored and redirected toward EUS monitoring. Only for the final step of stent deployment is the echoendoscope slightly withdrawn to obtain an endoscopic view[8,23] for control of the deployment of the intraluminal end of the transmural stent, a process demanding greater care than stent deployment at ERCP. The EUS scope is gently removed (approximately 2–3 cm) by an assistant in careful coordination with the endoscopist, who is simultaneously advancing the stent-delivery catheter under fluoroscopy and endoscopy, so as to maintain the half-deployed stent at the exact (fluoroscopic) point inside the duct where it was before scope withdrawal began. The intraluminal (GI) end of a transmural metal stent should be at least 2 cm in length, much longer than in standard transpapillary placement at ERCP. This point is of critical importance, because most metal stents foreshorten (up to 30% in some cases) during complete radial expansion, which takes hours. If the intraluminal segment is shorter than 2 cm, the stent may foreshorten toward the duct beyond the GI wall, resulting in free intraperitoneal or retroperitoneal leakage hours or days after placement.[33] Other approaches to stabilizing metal-stent position include forced balloon-assisted stent expansion immediately following initial stent deployment, which aims to control the otherwise blind process of natural stent expansion; or placement of a 7F double-pigtail stent inside the metal stent to safeguard against postprocedure dislocation and late migration.

Thus, the nuances of metal-stent expansion and foreshortening, the actual distance between the ultrasound transducer and the echoendoscope lens, and the potential for the virtual space between the GI wall and the target duct becoming a real space, explain why despite ductal access distances measuring less than 2 cm, metal stents of 6 cm or longer should be used. Shorter metal stents, despite looking adequate immediately after initial deployment, are prone to dislocation (foreshortening and/or migration) after the procedure. When these tedious technical tips are observed, transmural metal stenting provides immediate large-caliber drainage, with the advantage of a more effective sealing of the fistulous track than with use of plastic stents.[32,34] For additional details regarding the various steps involved in ESCP, the reader is referred to a recent review article.[23]

SUMMARY OF PUBLISHED LITERATURE

Biliary ESCP has been reported in around 400 cases, whereas approximately only 130 pancreatic ESCP procedures have been reported. **Table 1** summarizes results of published series with at least 10 biliary ESCP patients,[10,12–16,22,28,33,35–38] and pancreatic ESCP series[11,15,29,39,40] are summarized in **Table 2**. The preponderance of biliary versus pancreatic cases likely reflects multiple factors. First, biliary obstruction is a more common and more pressing clinical problem than pancreatic duct obstruction. Second, the technical challenges in accessing the main pancreatic duct through a hard, fibrotic pancreatic parenchyma, and successfully negotiating a guide wire through a tortuous duct with many side branches, are much greater than those involved in biliary ESCP. Third, the risks involved in pancreatic ESCP appear to be greater than those of biliary ESCP.[40] Finally, just as the clinical outcomes of pancreatic ERCP are somewhat less favorable than those of biliary ERCP, the clinical end point for biliary ESCP can be

Table 1
Results from series with more than 10 patients on bile duct drainage by ESCP

Authors,[Ref.] Year	n	Access		Technical Success		Drainage				Complications	
						Transpapillary		Transmural			
		IH	EH	n	(%)	RV	AG	HGS[a]	CDS[b]	n	(%)
Bories et al,[33] 2007	11	11	—	10	(91)	—	—	10	—	4	(36)
Horaguchi et al,[35] 2009	16	8	8	16	(100)	—	—	8	8	2	(12)
Brauer et al[28] 2009	12	—	12	11	(92)	7[c]	—	—	4	2	(16)
Maranki et al,[10] 2009	49	35	14	41	(84)	17[d]	17	3	4	8	(16)
Kim et al,[12] 2010	15	—	15	12	(80)	12	—	—	—	2	(13)
Hara et al,[36] 2011	18	—	18	17	(94)	—	—	—	17	3	(17)
Ramirez-Luna et al,[37] 2011	11	2	9	10	(91)	—	—	2	8	2	(18)
Fabbri et al,[14] 2011	16	—	16	12	(75)	3	—	—	9	1	(6)
Park et al,[16] 2011	57	31	26	55	(96)	2	—	26	27	11	(20)
Shah et al,[15] 2012	68	46[e]	12	58	(85)	39	10	8	1	6	(9)
Iwashita et al[13] 2012	40	9	31	29	(73)	29	—	—	—	5	(13)
Dhir et al,[22] 2012	58	—	58	57	(98)	57	—	—	—	2	(3)
Total	371	140	231	328	(88)	166	27	57	78	48	(13)

Whenever there is more than one report from same institution, only the latest one is included in the table.

Abbreviations: AG, antegrade; CDS, choledochoduodenostomy; EH, extrahepatic; HGS, hepaticogastrostomy; IH, intrahepatic; RV, rendezvous.

a Variant IH transmural drainage techniques also tallied under HGS (eg, hepaticojejunostomy in patients with total gastrectomy).

b Variant EH transmural drainage techniques also tallied under CDS (eg, choledochogastrostomy).

c Includes 4 true RV plus 3 retrograde non-RV, so-called road-map technique.

d Type of transpapillary drainage not stated. For the final tally in the table, out of 34 reported transpapillary drainage procedures, it was arbitrarily assumed that 50% were RV and 50% AG.

e Type of access not stated. For the final tally, a 1:4 ratio EH/IH was assumed based on prior published data from the group[38] and their explicit preference for IH access.

Table 2
Results from series with more than 10 patients on pancreatic duct drainage by ESCP

Authors,[Ref.] Year	n	Technical Success		Drainage				Complications	
				Transpapillary		Transmural			
		n	(%)	RV	non-RV[a]	PGS	PDS	n	(%)
Tessier et al,[11] 2007	36	33	(92)	—	—	26	7	5	(13)
Kahaleh et al,[39] 2007	13	10	(77)	—	—	10[b]	—	2	(15)
Will et al,[40] 2007	12	9	(77)	4	—	5	—	5	(42)
Barkay et al,[29] 2010	21	10	(48)	4	6	—	—	2	(10)
Shah et al,[15] 2012	22	19	(86)	9	—	10	—	4	(18)
Total	104	81	(78)	17	6	51	7	18	(17)
				23		58			

Whenever there is more than one report from same institution, only the latest one is included in the table.

Abbreviations: PDS, pancreaticoduodenostomy; PGS, pancreaticogastrostomy; RV, rendezvous.

[a] Non-RV transpapillary drainage refers to the methylene-blue pancreatography technique.

[b] All 10 patients had PGS, but in 7 of them the pancreaticogastric stent bridged also the papilla, thus also providing antegrade transpapillary drainage, whereas only 3 had standard PGS.

discerned more readily and more objectively than for pancreatic ESCP. These factors are reflected in the relative clinical success and complication rates for biliary (mean 88% success and 13% complications) versus pancreatic (mean 78% success and 17% complications) ESCP (see **Tables 1** and **2**). Whereas biliary ESCP is gradually gaining acceptance in many tertiary endoscopy units, pancreatic ESCP remains confined to very select units with special expertise in pancreatic endotherapy.

Most patients treated with ESCP had malignant biliary obstruction not amenable to standard ERCP palliation; only a relatively small number of patients had benign disease. This clinical profile probably reflects the greater anatomic distortion associated with malignancy, and the fact that surgery may be a more appealing salvage therapy after failed ERCP in operative candidates with benign strictures or CBD stones and in situ gallbladders.

Morbidity from ESCP is an important consideration. Complications arise from 2 sources: breach of the integrity of the duct and GI walls, inherent to all ESCP approaches, and trauma to the papilla. Breach of transluminal integrity is minimal in cases where just duct needle puncture is used (ie, rendezvous) and maximal where transmural drainage is performed (ie, CDS, HGS, or pancreaticogastrostomy). Breach may lead to leakage of intraperitoneal or retroperitoneal bile or pancreatic juice, ranging in severity from mild self-limiting abdominal pain accompanied by elevated white blood cell counts (a clinical scenario often labeled as pneumoperitoneum by investigators), to biloma (sometimes requiring drainage), bile peritonitis (with free fluid on cross-sectional imaging), or pseudocyst. Postprocedure pancreatitis may be a consequence of prior failed ERCP, direct pancreatic duct puncture, or antegrade transpapillary instrumentation (ie, balloon dilation or metal-stent insertion) during biliary ESCP. Similarly, bleeding may arise from endoscopic sphincterotomy (in cases where the rendezvous approach is used), but severe bleeding most commonly arises from transmural needle instrumentation (eg, repeat transhepatic punctures during difficult intrahepatic access) or, more typically, cautery tract dilation. Use of a needle knife has been identified as the single most significant predictor of complications during biliary ESCP.[16]

Although the breach of transluminal integrity is considered minimal by some investigators during needle rendezvous, it should be also noted that when transmural bile duct drainage is sought during ESCP at the outset (ie, not as salvage of failed prior attempted rendezvous), and a fully covered metal stent is used, acute postprocedure complications have been remarkably low.[32,34] All other complications of upper GI endoscopy, in particular cardiopulmonary events, are possible.[28] Another source of acute severe complications (including death from bile peritonitis[41]) or late less severe symptom recurrence is accounted for by transmural stent migration, particularly in patients with transmural pancreatic plastic stents.[11]

ROLE OF ESCP IN CLINICAL PRACTICE

Given its long record of proven effectiveness and reliable ability to train new adopters, ERCP is expected to remain the primary endoscopic modality for treatment of biliary and pancreatic ductal diseases. Advances in ERCP techniques (wire-guided cannulation, needle-knife access) and ERCP devices (sphincterotomes, guide wires, pancreatic stents) have improved ERCP success rates, and it seems reasonable to anticipate further technical enhancements in ERCP in the future. Other less invasive or noninvasive imaging modalities (EUS, magnetic resonance cholangiopancreatography [MRCP]) have largely supplanted ERCP as a diagnostic test. However, while these advances have contributed to the evolved perspective of ERCP as a primarily therapeutic intervention, reducing the overall volume of ERCP procedures, there has been a proportional increase in the volume of ERCPs undertaken with therapeutic intent.[4] Thus, although ESCP may be a therapeutic option for biliary or pancreatic disorders in a small subset of cases requiring endoscopic (ERCP) intervention, an increased demand for therapeutic ERCP could portend a greater role for ESCP in situations where ERCP is not feasible.

ESCP should be considered in situations where conventional ERCP has been unsuccessful by an experienced operator, and there remains a compelling indication for pancreatico-biliary therapy. Most commonly, this indication is biliary decompression caused by malignant obstruction although, as already noted, benign conditions have been managed successfully with ESCP. Of the available published series reviewed for this article, rates of unsuccessful ERCP that prompted ESCP ranged between 2% and 5%. In patients with low-grade or transient biliary obstruction, complete imaging workup, including diagnostic EUS and MRCP, is warranted before proceeding to ESCP.[7,23] Similarly, patients undergoing ESCP for pancreatic disease are highly selected, based on both the anatomy (pancreatic duct dilation, transection, or fistula) and clinical grounds (intractable pain, recurrent pancreatitis). Given the lower threshold for ERCP, ESCP may not be justified for all patients in whom ERCP has been unsuccessful. The clinical threshold for ESCP should be similar to that for percutaneous biliary drainage, and noninvasive follow-up as opposed to aggressive repeat attempts at ductal access, is advisable in patients with mild symptoms and negative or inconclusive imaging workup. Furthermore, ESCP should not be used as a means of gaining ductal access in the setting of only moderately difficult cannulation. Although some investigators have speculated that ESCP may be a potentially less invasive option than ERCP[42,43] given the lesser degree of papilla manipulation with ESCP, this view underestimates the difficulty and risks of ESCP. The most difficult ERCP is likely preferable to the easiest ESCP. The anatomic problems precluding ERCP in the ESCP literature range from complex postoperative anatomy (Roux-en-Y, pancreaticoduodenectomy) and severe tumor infiltration with or without duodenal stenosis, to high-grade hilar strictures and complete duct transections. Patients with lesser degrees of difficulty may be better served by a repeat attempt at ERCP by a highly experienced pancreatic-biliary endoscopist. Due consideration should be given to formulating a backup plan such as percutaneous biliary drainage or surgery if ESCP is unsuccessful.

As for the endoscopist who performs ESCP, he or she should be experienced and proficient in both ERCP and pancreatic-biliary EUS, with familiarity in EUS-FNA, guidewire manipulation, and stent placement. At present, ESCP is performed predominantly at centers with a high level of expertise in ERCP and a low incidence of failed ERCP. Expertise in endosonography and ERCP would seem to be the most important prerequisites for performing ESCP. Given that such endoscopic expertise exists outside tertiary centers, recommendations based on operator expertise rather than on institutional stratum may be more appropriate and conducive to the wider dissemination of this technique. Currently, in most centers the standard-of-care approach to failed ERCP is percutaneous or surgical drainage. However, as elaborated in this article, ESCP may be a superior alternative for selected patients. A prospective, randomized, multicenter study that compared ESCP, percutaneous drainage, and surgical drainage would be required to provide a high level of evidence to support one modality over the others.

SUMMARY

ESCP is an innovative technique that combines technical aspects of EUS and ERCP to effect biliary and pancreatic duct drainage in a very select subset of patients for whom this cannot be accomplished by conventional ERCP. ESCP is a hybrid modality that requires facility in both EUS-FNA and therapeutic ERCP. It has matured significantly over the past decade to the point where in many centers it is increasingly replacing percutaneous transhepatic biliary drainage for palliation of malignant obstructive jaundice after failed ERCP. Its role in managing anatomically complex chronic/relapsing pancreatitis is less well defined, but is based on the same technical grounds as biliary ESCP and the same clinical grounds as pancreatic ERCP. The many possible variant ESCP approaches are largely determined by patients' anatomy and to a lesser degree by operator preference. Careful planning and attention to minute details concerning needles, guide wires, dilators, and stents are advisable for every case. While high expectations are placed on the development of new devices to simplify ESCP in the future, they should not obscure the fact that ESCP has a significant learning curve and the potential for technical failure and complications. However, ESCP can successfully provide adequate therapy to very challenging patients in a minimally invasive fashion, and its use is expected to grow in clinical practice with the increasing availability of trained operators in both EUS and ERCP.

REFERENCES

1. Carr-Locke DL. Overview of the role of ERCP in the management of diseases of the biliary tract and the pancreas. Gastrointest Endosc 2002;56:S157–60.
2. van Delden OM, Lameris JS. Percutaneous drainage and stenting for palliation of malignant bile duct obstruction. Eur Radiol 2008;18:448–56.
3. Sohn TA, Lillemoe KD, Cameron JL, et al. Surgical palliation of unresectable periampullary adenocarcinoma in the 1990s. J Am Coll Surg 1999;188:658–66.
4. Martin JA. EUS-assisted ERP: throw me a line or just point out the way? Gastrointest Endosc 2010;71:1174–7.
5. Wiersema MJ, Sandusky D, Carr R, et al. Endosonography-guided cholangiopancreatography. Gastrointest Endosc 1996;43:102–6.
6. Giovannini M, Moutardier V, Pesenti C, et al. Endoscopic ultrasound-guided bilioduodenal anastomosis: a new technique for biliary drainage. Endoscopy 2001; 33:898–900.
7. Shami VM, Kahaleh M. Endoscopic ultrasonography (EUS)-guided access and therapy of pancreatico-biliary disorders: EUS-guided cholangio and pancreatic drainage. Gastrointest Endosc Clin N Am 2007;17:581–93, viii.
8. Will U, Meyer F. Endoscopic ultrasound-guided cholangiodrainage. In: Mönkemüller K, Wilcox CM, Muñoz-Navas M, editors. Interventional and therapeutic gastrointestinal endoscopy, vol. 27. Basel (Switzerland): Karger; 2010. p. 522–39.
9. Varadarajulu S, Tamhane A, Blakely J. Graded dilation technique for EUS-guided drainage of peripancreatic fluid collections: an assessment of outcomes and complications and technical proficiency (with video). Gastrointest Endosc 2008;68:656–66.
10. Maranki J, Hernandez AJ, Arslan B, et al. Interventional endoscopic ultrasound-guided cholangiography: long-term experience of an emerging alternative to percutaneous transhepatic cholangiography. Endoscopy 2009;41:532–8.
11. Tessier G, Bories E, Arvanitakis M, et al. EUS-guided pancreatogastrostomy and pancreatobulbostomy for the treatment of pain in patients with pancreatic ductal dilatation inaccessible for transpapillary endoscopic therapy Gastrointest Endosc 2007;65:233–41.
12. Kim YS, Gupta K, Mallery S, et al. Endoscopic ultrasound rendezvous for bile duct access using a transduodenal approach: cumulative experience at a single center. A case series. Endoscopy 2010;42:496–502.

13. Iwashita T, Lee JG, Shinoura S, et al. Endoscopic ultrasound-guided rendezvous for biliary access after failed cannulation. Endoscopy 2012;44:60–5.

14. Fabbri C, Luigiano C, Fuccio L, et al. EUS-guided biliary drainage with placement of a new partially covered biliary stent for palliation of malignant biliary obstruction: a case series. Endoscopy 2011;43:438–41.

15. Shah JN, Marson F, Weilert F, et al. Single-operator, single-session EUS-guided anterograde cholangiopancreatography in failed ERCP or inaccessible papilla. Gastrointest Endosc 2012;75:56–64.

16. Park DH, Jang JW, Lee SS, et al. EUS-guided biliary drainage with transluminal stenting after failed ERCP: predictors of adverse events and long-term results. Gastrointest Endosc 2011;74:1276–84.

17. Artifon EL, Safatle-Ribeiro AV, Ferreira FC, et al. EUS-guided antegrade transhepatic placement of a self-expandable metal stent in hepatico-jejunal anastomosis. JOP 2011;12:610–3.

18. Park DH, Jang JW, Lee SS, et al. EUS-guided transhepatic antegrade balloon dilation for benign bilioenteric anastomotic strictures in a patient with hepaticojejunostomy. Gastrointest Endosc 2012;75:692–3.

19. Gupta K, Mallery S, Hunter D, et al. Endoscopic ultrasound and percutaneous access for endoscopic biliary and pancreatic drainage after initially failed ERCP. Rev Gastroenterol Disord 2007;7:22–37.

20. Mallery S, Matlock J, Freeman ML. EUS-guided rendezvous drainage of obstructed biliary and pancreatic ducts: report of 6 cases. Gastrointest Endosc 2004;59:100–7.

21. Kahaleh M, Yoshida C, Kane L, et al. Interventional EUS cholangiography: a report of five cases. Gastrointest Endosc 2004;60:138–42.

22. Dhir V, Bhandari S, Bapat M, et al. Comparison of EUS-guided rendezvous and precut papillotomy techniques for biliary access (with videos). Gastrointest Endosc 2012;75:354–9.

23. Perez-Miranda M, De la Serna C, Diez-Redondo P, et al. Endosonography-guided cholangiopancreatography as a salvage drainage procedure for obstructed biliary and pancreatic ducts. World J Gastrointest Endosc 2010;2:212–22.

24. Kahaleh M, Wang P, Shami VM, et al. EUS-guided transhepatic cholangiography: report of 6 cases. Gastrointest Endosc 2005;61:307–13.

25. Kinney TP, Li R, Gupta K, et al. Therapeutic pancreatic endoscopy after Whipple resection requires rendezvous access. Endoscopy 2009;41:898–901.

26. Ryou M, Mullady DK, Dimaio CJ, et al. Pancreatic antegrade needle-knife (PANK) for treatment of symptomatic pancreatic duct obstruction in Whipple patients (with video). Gastrointest Endosc 2010;72:1081–8.

27. Dickey W. Parallel cannulation technique at ERCP rendezvous. Gastrointest Endosc 2006;63:686–7.

28. Brauer BC, Chen YK, Fukami N, et al. Single-operator EUS-guided cholangiopancreatography for difficult pancreaticobiliary access (with video). Gastrointest Endosc 2009;70:471–9.

29. Barkay O, Sherman S, McHenry L, et al. Therapeutic EUS-assisted endoscopic retrograde pancreatography after failed pancreatic duct cannulation at ERCP. Gastrointest Endosc 2010;71:1166–73.

30. Yamao K. EUS-guided choledochoduodenostomy. Gastrointest Endosc 2009;69:S194–9.

31. Tarantino I, Barresi L, Repici A, et al. EUS-guided biliary drainage: a case series. Endoscopy 2008;40:336–9.

32. Park DH, Koo JE, Oh J, et al. EUS-guided biliary drainage with one-step placement of a fully covered metal stent for malignant biliary obstruction: a prospective feasibility study. Am J Gastroenterol 2009;104:2168–74.
33. Bories E, Pesenti C, Caillol F, et al. Transgastric endoscopic ultrasonography-guided biliary drainage: results of a pilot study. Endoscopy 2007;39:287–91.
34. Park DH, Song TJ, Eum J, et al. EUS-guided hepaticogastrostomy with a fully covered metal stent as the biliary diversion technique for an occluded biliary metal stent after a failed ERCP (with videos). Gastrointest Endosc 2010;71:413–9.
35. Horaguchi J, Fujita N, Noda Y, et al. Endosonography-guided biliary drainage in cases with difficult transpapillary endoscopic biliary drainage. Dig Endosc 2009; 21:239–44.
36. Hara K, Yamao K, Niwa Y, et al. Prospective clinical study of EUS-guided choledochoduodenostomy for malignant lower biliary tract obstruction. Am J Gastroenterol 2011;106:1239–45.
37. Ramirez-Luna MA, Tellez-Avila FI, Giovannini M, et al. Endoscopic ultrasound-guided biliodigestive drainage is a good alternative in patients with unresectable cancer. Endoscopy 2011;43:826–30.
38. Nguyen-Tang T, Binmoeller KF, Sanchez-Yague A, et al. Endoscopic ultrasound (EUS)-guided transhepatic anterograde self-expandable metal stent (SEMS) placement across malignant biliary obstruction. Endoscopy 2010;42:232–6.
39. Kahaleh M, Hernandez AJ, Tokar J, et al. EUS-guided pancreaticogastrostomy: analysis of its efficacy to drain inaccessible pancreatic ducts. Gastrointest Endosc 2007;65:224–30.
40. Will U, Fueldner F, Thieme AK, et al. Transgastric pancreatography and EUS-guided drainage of the pancreatic duct. J Hepatobiliary Pancreat Surg 2007; 14:377–82.
41. Martins FP, Rossini LG, Ferrari AP. Migration of a covered metallic stent following endoscopic ultrasound-guided hepaticogastrostomy: fatal complication. Endoscopy 2010;42(Suppl 2):E126–7.
42. Puspok A, Lomoschitz F, Dejaco C, et al. Endoscopic ultrasound guided therapy of benign and malignant biliary obstruction: a case series. Am J Gastroenterol 2005;100:1743–7.
43. Savides TJ, Varadarajulu S, Palazzo L. EUS 2008 Working Group document: evaluation of EUS-guided hepaticogastrostomy. Gastrointest Endosc 2009;69:S3–7.

Endoscopic Management of Benign Biliary Strictures

Calvin H.Y. Chan, MBBS, FRACP, Jennifer J. Telford, MD, MPH, FRCPC*

KEYWORDS

- ERCP - Bile duct diseases - Pancreatitis - Cholangitis

KEY POINTS

- Specific techniques including multiple stent placement and the wide use of balloon dilatation have improved outcomes of biliary strictures, but many patients still require definitive surgical therapy for long-term success.
- The questions raised in the last 10 years regarding use of self-expandable metal biliary stents (SEMS) in benign disease have not yet been adequately addressed, but this will likely become clearer in the near future.
- New covered SEMS designs are awaited, along with the broader use of ancillary devices, including cholangioscopy, endoscopic ultrasound, and confocal microendoscopy, as well as new techniques in cytopathology to definitively exclude malignancy.
- Despite its limitations, the safety profile of endoscopic therapy still justifies its place as a first-line management option in benign biliary strictures.

 Video of a plastic biliary stent exchange in a patient with a benign distal biliary stricture secondary to chronic pancreatitis accompanies this article.

INTRODUCTION

Benign biliary strictures arise from a heterogeneous group of disorders with expansive causes, and a variable natural history. **Box 1** lists the common causes for benign biliary strictures. Postoperative and inflammatory strictures are the most common. The underlying causal factors usually involve local inflammation or ischemia and secondary fibrosis and scarring. Endoscopic retrograde cholangiopancreatography (ERCP) has usurped surgery as an established first-line diagnostic and therapeutic tool for most presentations of biliary strictures. Despite significant advances in endoscopic techniques and equipment, differentiating malignant from benign strictures can still be challenging; this is particularly relevant for patients with primary sclerosing

Division of Gastroenterology, St Paul's Hospital, The University of British Columbia, Vancouver, Canada
* Corresponding author. Pacific Gastroenterology Associates, 770-1190 Hornby Street, Vancouver, BC, Canada V6Z 2K5.
E-mail address: jtelford@telus.net

Gastrointest Endoscopy Clin N Am 22 (2012) 511–537
doi:10.1016/j.giec.2012.05.005
1052-5157/12/$ – see front matter Crown Copyright © 2012 Published by Elsevier Inc. All rights reserved.

| Box 1 |
| Causes of benign biliary strictures |

Postoperative causes

   Cholecystectomy

   Hepatic resection

   Biliary anastomosis

   Liver transplantation

   Biliary reconstruction

   Biliary: enteric anastomosis

Inflammatory

   Chronic pancreatitis and pseudocyst

   PSC

   Choledocholithiasis

   Immunoglobulin (Ig) G4 cholangiopathy

   Infections (recurrent bacterial cholangitis, tuberculosis, histoplasmosis, schistosomiasis, human immunodeficiency virus [HIV], parasites)

   Postradiation therapy

Other

   Ischemic (hypotension, hepatic artery thrombosis, portal biliopathy)

   Trauma

   Mirizzi syndrome

   Postbiliary sphincterotomy

cholangitis (PSC). In addition, some causes such as chronic pancreatitis remain resistant to endoscopic therapy. This article focuses on the endoscopic management of benign biliary strictures, discusses the general principles, and elaborates on optimal treatment strategies for the more common causes.

GENERAL PRINCIPLES
Diagnosis

Biliary strictures are usually diagnosed based on signs and symptoms of biliary obstruction (abnormal liver function tests, jaundice, abdominal pain, and cholangitis) and evidence of biliary dilatation on imaging. A detailed history to identify risk factors for differing causes should be sought. Localization of the stricture can be guided by cross-axial imaging and identifying a transition point to dilatation. Confirmation of the stricture ultimately depends on cholangiography, either contrast-enhanced or magnetic resonance cholangiopancreatography (MRCP). The modality of imaging used depends on the clinical presentation, the availability and expertise of available investigations at the medical institution, and the clinical suspicion for a stricture at presentation. If a proximal stricture (hilar or intrahepatic ducts) is suspected, cross-axial imaging is preferred before ERCP because other interventions aside from ERCP may be required. For patients with PSC, an MRCP before ERCP is advisable to ensure that instrumentation and subsequent contamination of the biliary tree is appropriate.

Exclude Malignancy

An accurate assessment of the cause and anatomic location of the stricture is critical to gauge success in endoscopic management. Malignancy should always be considered and tissue sampling performed at the initial and subsequent ERCPs. This sampling is usually performed via biliary epithelial tissue brushings or, less commonly, biopsy using a duodenoscope or cholangioscope. The sensitivity and specificity of bile duct brushings ranges from 35% to 70% and 90% respectively.[1,2] Brushings obtained after dilatation have not consistently been proved to increase yield.[3,4] Endoscopic ultrasound (EUS) and fine needle aspiration (FNA) are also useful in the evaluation of a biliary stricture as discussed later.

Stricture Characteristics

The location and length of the stricture can be helpful in determining the underlying cause, and guiding the technical considerations of management. Long strictures are more suspicious of a malignant process. Distal biliary strictures can be related to disorders in the pancreatic head. Hilar strictures are concerning for cholangiocarcinoma or an iatrogenic process. Diffuse stricturing and sclerosis is concerning for a systemic inflammatory or infective cause.

Classification

Anatomic classification guides optimal management strategy. Classification systems for benign strictures have been adapted from postoperative stricture findings. The Bismuth classification is the most commonly adapted system used and is based on stricture location and relationship to the confluence.[5] The Bismuth classifications of malignant and benign stricture differ (**Table 1**).[5,6] The Strasberg classification (**Table 2**) is based on location, size, and bile leakage.[7] Hilar and intrahepatic strictures are technically more challenging for the endoscopist, and additional measures including percutaneous transhepatic cholangiography (PTC) may be required for management. In Bismuth IV strictures involving both left and right ducts, endoscopic

Table 1
Bismuth classification of benign and malignant strictures

Classification	Benign Disease	Malignant Disease
I	Low CHD stricture, >2 cm distal to hilum	Tumor distal to the hepatic confluence
II	Proximal CHD stricture, <2 cm distal to hilum	Tumor involving hepatic confluence but preserved left and right duct communication
III	Hilar involvement up to proximal extent of CHD, but confluence preserved	Tumor involves CHD with right (IIIa) and left (IIIb) hepatic duct involvement
IV	Confluence involved, no communication between left and right ducts	Multicentric with right and left hepatic duct involvement
V	Type I, II, or III plus stricture of an isolated (aberrant) right duct	—

Abbreviation: CHD, common hepatic duct.
Data from Bismuth H. Postoperative strictures of the biliary tract. In: Blumgart L, editor. The biliary tract clinical surgery international. Edinburgh: Churchill Livingstone; 1982. p. 209–18; and Bismuth H, Nakache R, Diamond T. Management strategies in resection for hilar cholangiocarcinoma. Ann Surg 1992;215:31–8.

Table 2	
Strasberg classification for benign biliary strictures	
Class	**Injury Type**
A	Small duct injury in continuity with biliary system, with cystic duct leak
B	Injury to sectoral duct with consequent obstruction
C	Injury to sectoral duct with consequent bile leak from a duct not in continuity with biliary system
D	Injury lateral to extrahepatic ducts
E1	Stricture located >2 cm from bile duct confluence
E2	Stricture located <2 cm from the bile duct confluence
E3	Stricture located at bile duct confluence
E4	Stricture involving right and left bile ducts
E5	Complete occlusion of all bile ducts

Data from Strasberg SM, Hertl M, Soper NJ. An analysis of the problem of biliary injury during laparoscopic cholecystectomy. J Am Coll Surg 1995;180:101–25.

drainage of both lobes is not always possible. It is critical to ascertain which segments will benefit most from drainage. The right lobe typically drains most of the liver and decompressing the right hepatic duct usually provides more clinical benefit. Assessing for lobar atrophy on imaging may also guide management decisions.

ERCP
Technique

Benign biliary strictures often require multiple endoscopic sessions before complete and sustained resolution is deemed a success or failure. Failure rates are high in particular subgroups. Medical and surgical options should always be considered as adjunct or salvage therapy before and during the course of endoscopic therapy.

From the time a stricture is identified, the primary aims of management include biliary decompression to prevent secondary complications; identification of the underlying cause, with a focus on exclusion of malignancy; and anticipation for adjunct or rescue therapies should endoscopic therapy not succeed. For patients who may require definitive surgical management (liver transplantation, partial hepatectomy, Whipple procedure, or biliary bypass surgery), endoscopic management should be used as bridging therapy and focus should be on optimizing surgical success.

After biliary cannulation is achieved, guidewire choice, the need for dilatation, and stent choice are the 3 main technical decisions to consider. A guidewire should traverse the stricture to secure access, and 1 or several stents placed across the stricture with or without dilatation. Cytology should be obtained to exclude malignancy. In general, the maximum number of stents possible placed side by side should be inserted. A biliary sphincterotomy is recommended to ensure biliary access on subsequent ERCPs. The duration of endoscopic therapy should be 12 months before it is deemed unsuccessful (Video 1).

Guidewire Passage

Guidewires are critical in maintaining biliary access, directing the catheter and stent into the correct segment, and can aid in minimizing contrast contamination of the biliary tree. In a small proportion of patients, it can be difficult to traverse the stricture because of the severity of stenosis. There are many guidewires available with different characteristics, but few comparative studies are available to guide choice of wire in traversing difficult strictures. Early studies found hydrophilic wires to be more successful in cannulation across strictures compared with traditional monofilament wires.[8,9] Factors to consider in wire choice include construction material, tip characteristics, and diameter. Wire tips can be straight, tapered, J shaped, or looped; however, there is a paucity of literature to support their design goals.[10]

Stent Choice

Plastic stents are still the stent of choice for most benign conditions, but there are multiple studies being undertaken assessing self-expandable metal biliary stents (SEMS). Although many studies comparing different plastic stents were designed with malignant biliary obstruction, stents characteristics are extrapolated to the benign cohort. Stent characteristics vary in their construction material, length, angulation, and antimigration properties. Polyethylene flanged stents were first introduced more than 20 years ago and have survived the test of time despite attempts to improve on their longevity. Both Teflon and hydrophilic polymer-coated polyurethane (HPCP) materials have been compared with polyethylene. Van Berkel and colleagues[11] first compared Teflon with polyethylene stents and found no difference in duration of patency. HPCP was initially thought to reduce biofilm formation with its lower friction coefficient and hydrophilic property, but van Berkel and colleagues[12] found a shorter patency period in the HPCP group. The Tannenbaum stent (Cook UK, Letchworth, Hertfordshire, UK) was designed to improve longevity by eliminating side holes and changing stent material from polyethylene to Teflon, with 3 prospective studies failing to identify superiority, and raising concerns about higher migration rates.[13–15] Dietary fibers have been confirmed to fill the lumen of biliary stents to contribute to occlusion; however, addition of an antireflux valve (Fusion Marathon, Cook Inc., Winston, Salem, NC, USA)[16,17] has yet to prove advantageous. More recently, another novel stent construction limiting the central lumen by using a winged perimeter star-shaped design (Viaduct stent, GI Supply, Camp Hill, PA, USA)[18] has been introduced into the market (**Fig. 1**). As yet, there are no studies comparing this design with the traditional stents but the authors have a protocol under review for a randomized trial comparing the polyethylene stent with the Viaduct stent, with results anticipated in 2013.

Metal Biliary Stents

Interest continues in SEMS in the treatment of benign disease. It has theoretic advantages in terms of a narrow deployment system, innate expansile force minimizing the

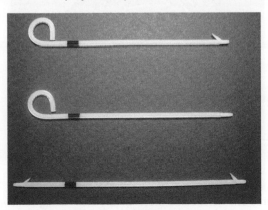

Fig. 1. Viaduct (GI Supply, Camp Hill, PA, USA) biliary stents.

need for dilatation, and a larger postdeployment diameter to minimize occlusion and consequently the duration for stent change. Early studies on fully uncovered SEMS placed without the intention of subsequent removal had a high rate of occlusion at approximately 2 years. These stents are not recommended for benign disease because of problems with stent embedment making them hard to remove.[19–21] SEMS may be fully covered or partially covered with the proximal and distal ends bare. The latter are more difficult to remove because of tissue ingrowth at the uncovered ends (**Fig. 2**).[22,23] Most published SEMS studies have stent therapy with a duration of 2 to 6 months, and stricture resolution has ranged from 60% to 100% at the time of stent removal. Migration rates have varied between 10% and 40%, with most fully covered SEMS studies at the higher end of the range.[22–27] Another potential complication of SEMS in benign disease is secondary stricture formation.[22,28,29] In the next 5 years, we anticipate results from prospective studies with longer follow-up than what is presently published to provide clarity regarding SEMS selection and duration of therapy (ClinicalTrials.gov identifiers NCT01238900, NCT00945516, NCT01221311). Evaluation of new stent designs with anchoring flaps[30] or a variable contour (Niti-S bumpy-type stent, Taewoong Medical, Seoul, Korea) may overcome current concerns of migration. Several recent case reports have also described the use of combined metal and plastic stents in the management of hilar strictures[31] and to avoid stent migration.[32] **Table 3** outlines published trials on the use of metal biliary stents in benign disease.

Stricture Dilation

Strictures can be dilated using either a balloon or bougie system. There are no head-to-head comparisons between the 2 techniques. The degree of dilatation is guided by the size of the bile duct distal to the stricture. Anecdotally, balloon dilation of focal strictures has the advantage of showing a waist fluoroscopically, the persistence of which indicates a need for further dilatation (**Fig. 3**). Dilatation soon after biliary anastomosis can lead to dehiscence, so a more cautious approach is required in this setting.[33] Most strictures should be stented after dilatation, because recurrence rates of nearly 50% have been described with dilatation alone,[34] although this is not an absolute rule, and does depend on the underlying cause.

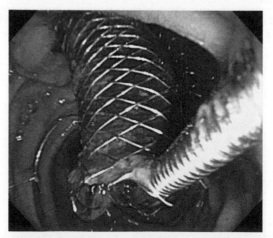

Fig. 2. A fully covered self-expandable metal biliary stent being removed using grasping forceps from a patient with a transplant anastomotic stricture.

Table 3
Metal biliary stents in benign biliary strictures

Study	Year	Number of Patients	Indication	Stent Type	Duration, Range (mo)	Follow-up Duration, Range (mo)	Result	Complication
Bruno et al[140,a]	2005	4	CP	FC (Hanaro, MI tech, Seoul, Korea)	3–6	Nil	75% stricture resolution	Proximal migration (1)
Tringali et al[141,a]	2005	6	CP	PC (not stated)	N/A	35 (33–37)	20-mo patency (range 16–24 mo)	Not reported
Cantu et al[23]	2005	14	CP	PC (Wallstent, Boston Scientific, Natick, MA)	21 (18–33)	22 (12–33)	50% stent dysfunction, median patency 21 mo (range 18–33 mo)	Cholangitis (5) Ingrowth (5) Distal migration (1) Proximal migration (1)
Kuo et al[142]	2006	3	OLT	FC (Viabil, WL Gore & Associates, Flagstaff, AZ)	38 d (0–49 d)	38 (0–49)	100% unremarkable cholangiogram at time of removal	Septicemia (1) Misplacement (1)
Kahaleh et al[22]	2008	79	CP (32), OLT (16), BS (24), I (4), PS (3)	PC (microvasive endoscopy, Boston Scientific, Natick MA)	4 (1–28)	12 (3–26)	Resolution: 77% CP, 94% OLT, 100% other, 90% success overall	Distal migration (2) Proximal migration (6) Bile leak (1) Stricture (6) Pain (2)
Cahen et al[143]	2008	6	CP	FC (Hanaro, MI tech Seoul, Korea)	3–6	28–36	66% resolution, 1 stricture recurrence at 6 mo	Stent embedment (2) Proximal migration (1)
Park et al[30]	2011	43	CP (11), BS (26), OLT (2), PS (4)	FC (MI Tech Seoul, and Standard Sci-Tech, Seoul, Korea)	4–6	3–5	84% resolution, 7 patients with recurrence	Proximal migration (1) Distal migration (6) Post-ERCP pancreatitis (6) Cholangitis (2)

Abbreviations: BS, biliary stone disease; CP, chronic pancreatitis; FC, fully covered self-expandable metal stent; I, inflammatory; N/A, not applicable; OLT, orthotopic liver transplantation; PC, partially covered self-expandable metal stent; PS, postsurgical.
  a Published in abstract form only.

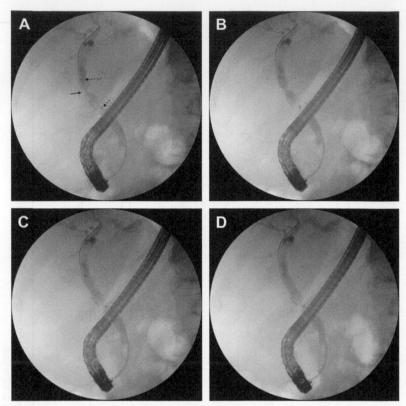

Fig. 3. Balloon dilatation of a posttransplant anastomotic stricture. (*A*) Initial cholangiogram showing stenosis at the anastomosis (*solid arrow*). The radio-opaque markings of the proximal and distal ends of a deflated balloon dilator are seen (*dashed arrows*). (*B* and *C*) Dilating balloon slowly inflated with gradual reduction in balloon waist. (*D*) Obliteration of balloon waste at conclusion of dilatation.

CHOLANGIOSCOPY

Cholangioscopy has a diagnostic usefulness in its ability to visualize and obtain tissue from the stricture. Its use is limited by the need for 2 endoscopists in most mother-daughter setups, endoscopist expertise, the need for extended procedure time, and cost of additional equipment.

Aside from targeted biopsies, the presence of dilated and tortuous vessels, otherwise termed capillary sign or tumor vessel sign, has been described to be highly specific for malignancy,[35,36] although subsequent studies have found benign stricture during the active inflammatory stage to mimic these vascular abnormalities.[37] Other cholangioscopic appearances associated with malignancy include friability and irregular surface.[38] Two studies found the sensitivity of cholangioscopy for diagnosing malignancy in indeterminate strictures to be more than 89%, but this was also associated with a higher false-positive rate with specificity as low as 86%.[37,39]

Therapeutic application of cholangioscopy in benign strictures is limited. There have been reports of cholangioscopy-assisted guidewire placement in strictures that were difficult to traverse,[40] but currently other techniques such as EUS-assisted cholangiography and guidewire placement or PTC-guided rendezvous remain more accessible options in most centers.

EUS

EUS compliments ERCP through its sonographic and tissue sampling capabilities. Although EUS with FNA of a visualized mass has a yield of approximately 90%,[41,42] FNA of biliary strictures in the absence of a mass is less rewarding. Studies of the diagnostic accuracy of EUS in excluding malignant biliary strictures have been limited by small sample size, differing gold standards, and often by a heterogeneous study population. FNA of distal biliary strictures has a higher diagnostic yield, perhaps because of its more intimate relationship to the transducer. Two studies assessing indeterminate strictures found the sensitivity of FNA alone to be less than 50%,[43,44] but, in 1 of the studies, sonographic features of a pancreatic head mass or irregular bile duct wall had a positive predictive value for malignancy of 100% and a negative predictive value of 84%.[44] Two meta-analyses on EUS with or without FNA for extrahepatic bile duct strictures have been performed. Inclusion criteria in both was broad, with 1 including gallbladder masses, and many studies were included before 1997. Pooled sensitivities were 0.78 and 0.84, and specificity was 0.84 and 1.00.[45,46]

From a therapeutic perspective, EUS can assist in stent placement if standard ERCP-guided transpapillary placement has failed, either in a rendezvous manner with ERCP, or by placing a stent in the biliary tree to traverse the stomach or duodenum.[47,48] This technique is challenging, partly because of the oblique view of the linear echoendoscope, and is still limited to experienced centers, but, as newer echoendoscopes become available, including a forward-viewing echoendoscope,[49] EUS may play a more prominent role in therapeutic biliary strictures.

INTRADUCTAL ULTRASOUND

Intraductal ultrasound has a sensitivity and specificity of between 80 and 90% in published studies in differentiating benign from malignant strictures.[48] It can identify echolayer disruption of the bile duct wall, as well as small adjacent mass lesions. Its use is limited by operator expertise, the often challenging imaging criteria for diagnosis, and the biliary contamination risk and subsequent need for ERCP and biliary stenting.[50,51] Where available, its role is most appropriate to patients with a high suspicion of malignancy when ERCP and EUS have both failed to prove malignancy.

CONFOCAL LASER ENDOMICROSCOPY

Probe-based confocal endomicroscopy has gained momentum as an emerging entity in its diagnostic usefulness in indeterminate biliary strictures. It uses a laser scanning unit to emit light and illuminate tissue. The light is absorbed by fluorophores, enhanced via intravenous fluorescein, and the reflected fluorescence is detected by the probe and optically relayed to the processing unit. This technique allows real-time histologic assessment of the target epithelium. The Miami classification for pancreaticobiliary strictures has recently been developed to standardize imaging features consistent with malignancy (**Table 4**). In a validation study involving 4 endoscopists and 41 patients, 5 of the 6 Miami criteria met acceptable interobserver variability with a κ value of more than 0.4.[52] New-generation probes have now been manufactured for compatibility with both the working channel of duodenoscopes and cholangioscopes. Published studies to date have described sensitivities of between 83% and 98%, specificities of 67% to 75%, and accuracy of 81% to 86%.[53,54] Further studies are required to validate and refine the diagnostic criteria and accuracy, address issues relating to training requirements, and confirm safety profile before it is ready to be endorsed into mainstream practice.

Table 4
Miami criteria for probe-based confocal endomicroscopy for predicting neoplasia in the pancreaticobiliary system

Suggestive for Malignancy	Suggestive for Benign Strictures
Thick, dark bands (>40 μm)	Thin, dark (branching) bands
Thick white bands (>20 μm)	Thin, white bands
Dark clumps	—
Epithelium visualized (villi, glands)	—
Fluorescein leakage	—

Data from Meining A, Shah RJ, Slivka A, et al. Classification of probe-based confocal laser endomicroscopy findings in pancreaticobiliary strictures. Endoscopy 2012;44(3):251–7; and Meining A, Chen YK, Pleskow D, et al. Direct visualization of indeterminate pancreaticobiliary strictures with probe-based confocal laser endomicroscopy: a multicenter experience. Gastrointest Endosc 2011;74:961–8.

MANAGEMENT OF SPECIFIC DISORDERS
Postoperative Benign Biliary Strictures

Postoperative benign biliary strictures occur most frequently after cholecystectomy, either as a consequence of direct ductal trauma (partial or complete transection by clipping or ligation) or ischemic insult from thermal or dissection injury. It is usually diagnosed 6 to 12 months after surgery, and earlier presentations can be associated with bile leak. In one of the earliest reported series on endoscopic management of bile duct complications after cholecystectomy, only half of the cohort developed abdominal pain and none were septic.[55]

The widespread application of laparoscopic approach to cholecystectomy has been associated with an increasing incidence of bile duct injuries. Estimated incidence has increased from approximately 0.1% to 0.2% to 0.4% to 0.6% compared with earlier studies in which open cholecystectomy was the mainstay of treatment.[56–58] Management of bile duct injuries has been predominantly surgical in the past. Although initial surgical success was reported to be more than 90%, follow-up studies have found a 9% to 25% recurrence rate, a morbidity rate of 40%, and a mortality of 1.3% to 1.7%.[56,59–61]

Endoscopic therapy has been associated with variable success, with reported response rates between 40% and 90%.[55,59,62–65] The diverse response rates are likely related to different intervals of patient follow-up after stent removal, because stricture recurrence can occur many months to years later. Two studies with a longer follow-up interval (median of 81 and mean of 23 months) reported a recurrence rate of 20% to 30% within 2 years.[64–66] Most published reviews are retrospective and include a heterogeneous cohort (some include transplant anastomotic strictures, some combine strictures and bile leak in analysis), variable and nonstandardized protocol (not all centers undertook rendezvous procedures), and variable follow-up and compliance. In 2 of the largest series, Bergman and colleagues[62] and Costamagna and colleagues[59] published retrospective studies in 2001 with long-term follow-up (mean of 9.1 years and 48.8 months respectively). Costamagna and colleagues[59] took a more aggressive approach to management by dilating and inserting the maximal number of stents possible and achieved a 76% completion rate with all but 1 case sustaining long-term relief, compared with only 47% in the study by Bergman and colleagues.[62]

Because of the limitations of high-quality evidence, the authors consider the following approach to management

- Endoscopic approach is a reasonable first line in patients suspected of having a postoperative biliary stricture, with an anticipated response rate of approximately 70%
- In patients with complete biliary obstruction in whom guidewire passage is difficult, we proceed to a rendezvous or surgical approach
- Biliary stenting should be performed for 6 to 18 months, with stent changes every 3 months
- Given the success rates of most studies deploying multiple stents, this approach is reasonable
- The need for universal stricture dilatation is unclear but is indicated if the endoscopist anticipates difficulty passing the stent across a stricture.

Transplant Biliary Strictures

Bile leaks and strictures are the most common biliary complications following liver transplantation. The incidence of posttransplant biliary strictures varies widely among different groups. In deceased donor transplants, the incidence is between 5% and 25%,[67–70] and up to 32% for living donor transplants.[71,72] Posttransplant biliary strictures are classified as anastomotic or nonanastomotic, and early (within 1 month) or late. Early strictures are generally related to perioperative events (excessive cautery, dissection, or tension of the duct anastomosis) and are mostly anastomotic. Late strictures are mainly caused by vascular insufficiency and fibrosis.[73,74] Several risk factors have been identified as being associated with posttransplant strictures, including the type of biliary anastomosis (Roux-en-Y choledochojejunostomy vs choledochocholedochostomy), the use of T tube (which is now less commonly used), hepatic artery thrombosis, prolonged warm and cold ischemia time, ABO incompatibility, use of donor after cardiac death, and posttransplant bile leak.[75–79] Accurate assessment of these subtypes helps guide the most appropriate course of management and predict likelihood of success.

Patients usually present with symptomatic or asymptomatic increase in liver function tests, but, unlike other causes of biliary obstruction, dilatation of the donor bile ducts is an unreliable indictor of biliary obstruction.[80] As such, cholangiography, whether it be noninvasive or invasive, is often required to diagnosis a stricture when the clinical suspicion arises. A Doppler of the hepatic vessels should be included in the initial assessment to exclude hepatic artery thrombosis. The choice of MRCP or a diagnostic ERCP is guided by local expertise and availability, as well as the pretest probability of requiring intervention. MRCP has a sensitivity and specificity of between 87% and 100% and a negative predictive value of more than 90% in diagnosing biliary strictures.[81,82] Scintigraphy has also been shown to have a high specificity but lower sensitivity for diagnosing bile duct strictures.[83]

Characteristic cholangiographic findings result from differing pathophysiology. Nonanastomotic strictures usually arise from biliary ischemia secondary to hepatic artery stenosis or thrombosis, because this is the sole blood supply to the biliary tree.[84] They typically occur at the hilum and can progress to the intrahepatic ducts, occasionally in multiple locations.[85] They typically occur earlier than anastomotic strictures, with a mean time to stricture development between 3 and 6 months.[86,87] Disease recurrence, especially PSC and infection, are other causes of nonanastomotic strictures.[87] Anastomotic stricture usually occurs secondary to fibrosis and is represented by a short focal stricture. Early anastomotic strictures can be a result of local edema and inflammation, which often resolves over a period of 2 to 3 months.

Endoscopic therapy is now widely recognized as the first-line management approach for posttransplant biliary strictures, with PTC and surgical bypass reserved for unsuccessful cases. In patients with Roux-en-Y anastomosis, ERCP may not be possible, and PTC with dilatation and catheter placement may be more appropriate. Retransplantation remains a final option if other therapies fail.

Anastomotic Strictures

Most anastomotic strictures arise within the first 12 months of transplantation (**Fig. 4**). Early anastomotic strictures, usually caused by edema and inflammation, have a good response to therapy and are less likely to recur, with resolution of stricture over an average of 3 months.[88,89] Delayed-onset anastomotic strictures, a consequence of fibrotic scarring, require a more protracted course of therapy. Most published studies have been retrospective, and the few prospective studies have been limited by small sample size and a heterogeneous cohort. Balloon dilatation to a maximal diameter of the duct up to 10 mm followed by insertion of multiple plastic stents decreases stricture recurrence by 62% to 31% compared with balloon dilatation alone.[90,91] Multiple published studies have shown that a protocol of balloon dilatation with 3-monthly stent changes with insertion of multiple side-by-side stents increases success to 80% to 90% (**Fig. 5**).[86,88,92,93] Treatment is usually maintained for 12 to 24 months before it is considered a failure.

There are 2 case series assessing SEMS in anastomotic strictures (**Fig. 6**, **Table 5**).[27,94] Preliminary reports are favorable enough to support further prospective evaluation. Manufacturers are currently developing SEMS that maximize stent removability and antimigratory and antiembedment properties.[95,96] There are currently at least 3 enrolled, prospective, randomized trials evaluating fully covered SEMS in the management of anastomotic strictures (ClinicalTrials.gov identifier NCT01151280, NCT01148199, and NCT01432808).

Nonanastomotic Strictures

Nonanastomotic strictures comprise 10% to 25% of transplant-related strictures, and tend to occur earlier than anastomotic strictures.[67,87] Response to endoscopic

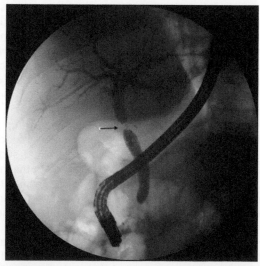

Fig. 4. Posttransplant anastomotic stricture with near-complete stenosis (*arrow*). Donor and native ducts are of a similar diameter.

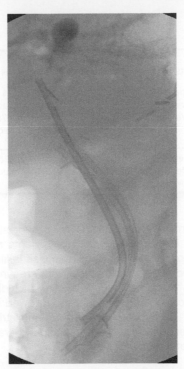

Fig. 5. Fluoroscopic image at the end of procedure after placement of 3 plastic biliary stents in a patient with a posttransplant anastomotic stricture.

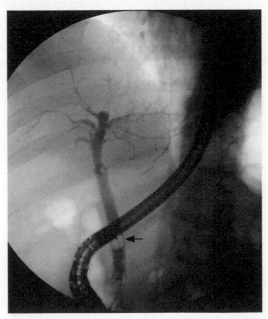

Fig. 6. A fully covered self-expandable metal stent about to be removed in a patient with a transplant anastomotic stricture. Note that an extraction balloon was used to obtain an occlusion cholangiogram (*arrow*) because of the patency of the biliary orifice as a result of the stent being in situ.

Table 5
Self-expandable metal stents for transplant anastomotic strictures

Chaput et al[27]	2010	22	Partially covered Wallstent	2 mo	12 mo	86% initial success, 47.4% recurrence	Pancreatitis = 3 Stent migration = 2 Cholangitis = 1 Pain = 1
Garcia-Pajares et al[94]	2010	22	Covered (details not specified)	Not specified	12.5 mo (median)	95.5% success	Migration = 5 Embedment = 1 Pain = 4

therapy is low, ranging from 0% to 50% in published studies, and treatment is usually more prolonged.[77,86,89,97] Up to 30% to 50% of patients require retransplantation despite endoscopic therapy.[33,73,86] The poor response is likely related to the multifocal stricture, associated sludge and casts, and recurrence of an underlying disorder.[87] The principles of therapy remain similar, including extraction of sludge and casts and dilatation of accessible strictures, followed by placement of plastic stents every 3 months.[89] Compared with anastomotic strictures, nonanastomotic strictures have a lower response rate to endoscopic therapy (80% vs 0%)[86] and require a longer duration of therapy (67 vs 185 days).[98]

CHRONIC PANCREATITIS

Common bile duct (CBD) strictures are thought to occur in 10% to 30% of patients with chronic pancreatitis.[99,100] Although inflammation during an acute attack may result in periductal edema and secondary obstruction, fibrotic stricturing from chronic inflammation is the usual cause of CBD strictures in these patients (**Fig. 7**). Patients can be asymptomatic, and the goals of biliary decompression are to prevent complications of jaundice, cholangitis, secondary biliary cirrhosis, and choledocholithiasis.[101]

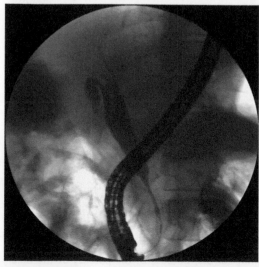

Fig. 7. Distal CBD stricture secondary to chronic pancreatitis.

Endoscopic therapy is a reasonable first-line and short-term management option; however, it tends to be less effective in treating strictures secondary to calcific pancreatitis and surgical bypass should always be considered if the patient is an appropriate surgical candidate and endoscopic therapy fails. Additional concerns of noncompliance to follow-up may sway the decision to surgery in this cohort.[102]

Cahen and colleagues[103] reported one of the largest cohorts of 58 patients who received a single 10-Fr stent with a median follow-up of 45 months. They found a 36% success rate with endoscopic treatment (24% in the group without concomitant acute pancreatitis). Stricture resolution was usually accomplished after 3 stent exchanges (reassessment at 12 months), without additional benefit with more prolonged treatment. This approach forms the basis of common management practice of a 12-month course of endoscopic therapy. All patients with a response remained stricture free.

In an effort to improve these results, Catalano and colleagues[98] enrolled 12 patients with the intention of inserting 5 stents (mean 4.3) and achieved a 92% response, although their definition of response was not clear. Although Catalano and colleagues[98] and others have noted that patients with calcific pancreatitis have a lower response rate, Pozsar and colleagues[104] reported a 62% success to multiple stent therapy in this group.

SEMS are increasing used in biliary strictures associated with chronic pancreatitis , but current literature is still limited, and response seems inferior to other benign causes. Initial studies assessed the role of metal stents as a permanent prosthesis to maintain biliary patency, but stent failure became a problem with longer follow-up intervals. Deviere and colleagues[20] prospectively followed 20 patients who underwent uncovered SEMS placement for a mean period of 33 months and maintained patency in 18 patients. Yamaguchi and colleagues[105] followed 8 patients who underwent uncovered SEMS placement to treat biliary strictures secondary to chronic pancreatitis for a minimum of 5 years. Complications occurred in 4 of 8 patients, but only after almost 5 years. Cantu and colleagues[23] similarly found a 50% stent failure rate when patients were followed for an additional 22 months. The temporary placement of covered SEMS has also been assessed. Studies presently focus on temporary placement of SEMS and assessment of patency, migration, and retrievability. Kahaleh and colleagues[22] reported a 77% response in their subgroup of 22 patients with biliary strictures secondary to chronic pancreatitis who underwent partially covered SEMS placement. This finding compared with a 90% response rate in the population of benign biliary strictures with a median of 12 months of stent therapy. SEMS migration occurred in 14% of patients and the investigators suggested that the duration of stent therapy should not exceed 6 months. A recently published abstract evaluated the long-term outcome in 121 patients who underwent fully or partially covered SEMS insertion for the management of benign bile duct strictures for a mean of 121 days. Successful stricture resolution was documented in 50% of patients with chronic pancreatitis, compared with 71% in bile duct strictures from any cause. Also concerning was a 20% complication rate including 16% migration.[106] The results of 2 prospective trials are awaited over the next few years (ClinicalTrials. gov identifiers NCT01085747 and NCT01457092).

At present, surgical bypass remains the most viable long-term option unless contraindications to surgery exist. The need for pancreatic or enteral bypass should be factored into the surgical decision. Changes in covered SEMS design that allow for longer duration of therapy without tissue ingrowth or stent migration are needed before SEMS can be used as standard practice in bile duct strictures secondary to chronic pancreatitis.

PSC

PSC is a chronic progressive inflammatory disorder affecting the medium and large intrahepatic and extrahepatic bile ducts. Because the stricturing process is diffuse, with most patients having intrahepatic and extrahepatic duct involvement **(Fig. 8)**,[107] endoscopic management focuses on treatment of dominant strictures. Between 15% and 60% of patients with PSC develop a dominant stricture.[108–110] The management of PSC with a dominant stricture is challenging on multiple fronts; the difficulty in distinguishing malignant from benign strictures, the difficulty in managing proximal and multiple strictures, the high rate of secondary bacterial cholangitis, and the lack of definitive therapeutic strategies aside from liver transplantation, are all critical factors in deciding the best path to management.

Malignancy always needs to be considered and excluded in the management of dominant strictures. The prevalence of cholangiocarcinoma in PSC ranges from around 8% to 25%.[111,112] In one of the earliest studies of ursodeoxycholic acid in PSC, 62% of patients who developed a cholangiocarcinoma had a dominant stricture.[113] Multiple studies have investigated the most accurate diagnostic modality for cholangiocarcinoma. Serum tumor markers including CA19-9 alone are inadequate for diagnosis, with sensitivities and specificities ranging from 14% to 42%.[114,115] Sensitivities of routine bile duct brushings have ranged from 29% to 73%, with generally high specificities.[114,116] More recently, fluorescent in situ hybridization (FISH) has been studied in cytology samples, with 2 chromosomal abnormalities observed: polysomy and trisomy of chromosomes 7 or 3. In 36 patients affected by PSC with cholangiocarcinoma, FISH was 64% sensitive, 70% specific, 68% accurate, and had positive and negative predictive values of 60% and 74%, respectively.[114] A more recent study found that 9 of 13 patients with serial polysomy were diagnosed with cholangiocarcinoma, in 4 of whom malignancy was not

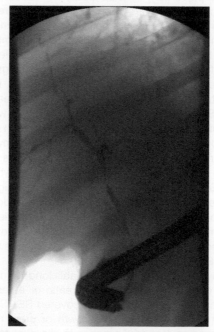

Fig. 8. Cholangiogram of a patient with PSC. Diffuse intrahepatic beading with a dominant common hepatic duct stricture is seen.

confirmed by other modalities until 1 to 3 years later.[117] More studies are required before FISH is used in mainstream practice.

ERCP and MRCP are the modalities of choice for diagnosis. ERCP is more sensitive than MRCP in detecting extrahepatic dominant strictures and early PSC,[118] and allows tissue sampling and therapeutic intervention.[119] However, its invasive nature and associated morbidity, with cholangitis rates of 10%[120] and overall complications of up to 50%,[121] have made MRCP an important first-line modality, with ERCP reserved only for therapeutic intent.

Management decisions should consider the impact on liver transplantation, the only cure for PSC. Progression of PSC is generally slow, and early management of dominant strictures should be designed to improve symptoms and quality of life without jeopardizing successful and timely transplant. Endoscopic biliary dilatation of dominant strictures, usually with multiple sessions, achieves clinical and biochemical response in around 80% of cases.[109,121,122] Several studies have shown a better predicted Mayo risk score after endoscopic therapy.[123–125] These studies were mainly observational, with endoscopic treatment combined with ursodeoxycholic acid, making it difficult to draw conclusions on endotherapy alone. One retrospective study found complication rates to be higher with stenting compared with dilatation alone,[126] which led Ponsioen and colleagues[127] to propose a short-term stenting protocol of 10 days that has reported success.

Most clinicians therefore perform biliary dilatation up to 24 Fr and apply a biliary stent to maintain patency, with administration of prophylactic antibiotics during and after the procedure. No prospective studies have compared the optimal duration of stent therapy with the frequency of endoscopic dilatation of dominant strictures. No studies have compared the endoscopic versus surgical therapies for dominant strictures.

IGG4 CHOLANGIOPATHY

IgG4 cholangiopathy or IgG4 sclerosing cholangitis remains an evolving clinical entity, with endoscopic management playing a supportive role to immunosuppressive therapy. It is a unique systemic inflammatory condition characterized by IgG4 plasma cell infiltration of various organs as well as high serum IgG4. Most patients with IgG4 cholangiopathy have associated autoimmune pancreatitis, and biliary obstruction can be from primary biliary inflammation or secondary to a pancreatic mass (**Fig. 9**). Diagnosis can be difficult and confused with PSC, especially in the absence of reliable histology and when IgG4 staining is not available (**Fig. 10**). Nakazawa and colleagues[128,129] proposed the use of cholangiographic characteristics to differentiate PSC from IgG4 cholangiopathy (beaded, prune tree, diverticulumlike, vs bandlike, segmental, and long stricture with prestenotic dilatation). The usefulness of these features was disputed in a 17-physician study comparing cholangiogram interpretation of PSC, cholangiocarcinoma, and IgG4 cholangiopathy, with interobserver agreement of only 0.18.[130]

Although response to corticosteroid therapy is less predictable than with pancreatic disease, medical therapy and immunosuppression remains the primary therapy. There is minimal literature describing endoscopic therapy for IgG4 cholangiopathy but, based on general principles, endoscopic stenting has a role to relieve jaundice during medical therapy.

HIV CHOLANGIOPATHY

HIV cholangiopathy is a rare condition, first described in the late 1980s, that is associated with cholangiographic abnormalities including papillary stenosis, sclerosing

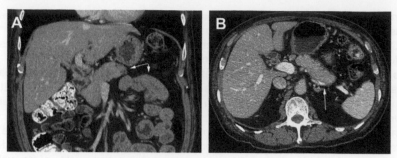

Fig. 9. (A, B) Computed tomography imaging of a patient with autoimmune pancreatitis. The pancreas appears bulky and sausagelike (arrows).

cholangitis, and biliary strictures. Extrahepatic biliary strictures alone or combined with intrahepatic duct strictures and papillary stenosis occur in approximately one-third of patients. It typically occurs in patients with CD4 counts less than $100/mm^3$, and is therefore an extremely rare entity in the current era of highly active antiretroviral therapy (HAART). HIV cholangiopathy is associated with chronic biliary tract infections, most commonly with *Cryptosporidium parvum* but also cytomegalovirus, *Microsporidium*, and *Cyclospora*.[131]

Because patients with HIV cholangiopathy have advanced disease with a short median survival, treatment is designed to control symptoms. Antimicrobial therapy does not generally improve symptoms or cholangiographic appearance. Endoscopic sphincterotomy is effective at relieving pain in patients with papillary stenosis.[131,132] Extrahepatic biliary strictures are managed with plastic stent therapy, whereas Castiella and colleagues[133] described response to ursodeoxycholic acid for intrahepatic sclerosis.

OTHER CAUSES OF BENIGN BILIARY STRICTURES

Ischemic cholangiopathy is most often related to compromise to the hepatic artery as a result of liver transplantation, but can occur in the setting of transarterial

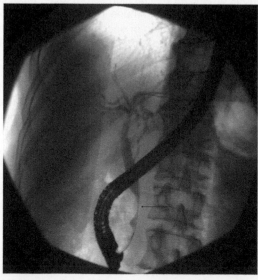

Fig. 10. Smooth distal CBD stricture (arrow) in a patient with autoimmune pancreatitis.

chemoembolization and radiotherapy, and rarely in hypercoagulable states. Thrombosis of the portal vein with secondary recanalization leads to engorgement of the 2 venous plexuses of the biliary tree, (epicholedochal venous plexus of Saint, and the paracholedochal veins of Petren), leading to extrinsic compression of the biliary tree and its supplying arterioles.[134] The resulting ischemia and fibrosis can lead to biliary strictures, otherwise known as portal biliopathy. Only a small proportion of patients with portal vein thrombosis develop biliary complications. Cholangiographic abnormalities include smooth strictures, undulations, caliber irregularities, and duct displacement. The CBD is more commonly involved than the intrahepatic ducts.[135,136] Because of the presence of multiple incomplete segments of biliary tract obstruction, patients are prone to stone formation and its associated complications. Case series have described a higher bleeding complication rate during endoscopic management caused by the presence of choledochal varices, and thrombocytopenia secondary to hypersplenism.[137] Extra care should be taken when performing sphincterotomy and extraction of stones to minimize mucosal and ductal trauma.

BILIARY-ENTERIC STRICTURES

Balloon-assisted enteroscopes have allowed endoscopic access to the biliary system in patients with surgically altered anatomy, with success rates of up to 75%.[138,139] Its use is still currently limited by expertise, lack of accompanying endoscopic accessories, and a higher risk of complications.

SUMMARY

In the last 20 years, endoscopic management of benign biliary strictures has been evolutionary rather than revolutionary. Although specific techniques including multiple stent placement and the wide use of balloon dilatation have improved outcomes, many patients still require definitive surgical therapy for long-term success. The questions raised in the last 10 years regarding the use of SEMS in benign disease have not been adequately addressed, although this will likely be clearer in the near future. New covered SEMS designs and broader use of ancillary devices are awaited, including cholangioscopy, EUS, and confocal microendoscopy, as well as new techniques in cytopathology to definitively exclude malignancy. Despite its limitations, the safety profile of endoscopic therapy still justifies its place as a first-line management option in benign biliary strictures.

ACKNOWLEDGMENTS

The authors thank Dr Urs Steinbrecher of the University of British Columbia for his contribution to **Figs. 2–6**.

SUPPLEMENTARY DATA

Supplementary data related to this article can be found online at doi:10.1016/j.giec. 2012.05.005.

REFERENCES

1. Kurzawinski TR, Deery A, Dooley JS, et al. A prospective study of biliary cytology in 100 patients with bile duct strictures. Hepatology 1993;18:1399–403.

2. Glasbrenner B, Ardan M, Boeck W, et al. Prospective evaluation of brush cytology of biliary strictures during endoscopic retrograde cholangiopancreatography. Endoscopy 1999;31:712–7.

3. de Bellis M, Fogel EL, Sherman S, et al. Influence of stricture dilation and repeat brushing on the cancer detection rate of brush cytology in the evaluation of malignant biliary obstruction. Gastrointest Endosc 2003;58:176–82.

4. Farrell RJ, Jain AK, Brandwein SL, et al. The combination of stricture dilation, endoscopic needle aspiration, and biliary brushings significantly improves diagnostic yield from malignant bile duct strictures. Gastrointest Endosc 2001;54:587–94.

5. Bismuth H. Postoperative strictures of the biliary tract. In: Blumgart L, editor. The biliary tract clinical surgery international. Edinburgh (UK): Churchill Livingstone; 1982. p. 209–18.

6. Bismuth H, Nakache R, Diamond T. Management strategies in resection for hilar cholangiocarcinoma. Ann Surg 1992;215:31–8.

7. Strasberg SM, Hertl M, Soper NJ. An analysis of the problem of biliary injury during laparoscopic cholecystectomy. J Am Coll Surg 1995;180:101–25.

8. Gane E, Lane M, Hamilton I. Use of an alternative guidewire system in endoscopic placement of biliary endoprosthesis. Endoscopy 1991;23:215–7.

9. McCarthy JH, Miller GL, Laurence BH. Cannulation of the biliary tree, cystic duct and gallbladder using a hydrophilic polymer-coated steerable guide wire. Gastrointest Endosc 1990;36:386–9.

10. Somogyi L, Chuttani R, Croffie J, et al. Guidewires for use in GI endoscopy. Gastrointest Endosc 2007;65:571–6.

11. van Berkel AM, Boland C, Redekop WK, et al. A prospective randomized trial of Teflon versus polyethylene stents for distal malignant biliary obstruction. Endoscopy 1998;30:681–6.

12. van Berkel AM, Bruno MJ, Bergman JJ, et al. A prospective randomized study of hydrophilic polymer-coated polyurethane versus polyethylene stents in distal malignant biliary obstruction. Endoscopy 2003;35:478–82.

13. Catalano MF, Geenen JE, Lehman GA, et al. "Tannenbaum" Teflon stents versus traditional polyethylene stents for treatment of malignant biliary stricture. Gastrointest Endosc 2002;55:354–8.

14. England RE, Martin DF, Morris J, et al. A prospective randomised multicentre trial comparing 10 Fr Teflon Tannenbaum stents with 10 Fr polyethylene Cotton-Leung stents in patients with malignant common duct strictures. Gut 2000;46:395–400.

15. van Berkel AM, Huibregtse IL, Bergman JJ, et al. A prospective randomized trial of Tannenbaum-type Teflon-coated stents versus polyethylene stents for distal malignant biliary obstruction. Eur J Gastroenterol Hepatol 2004;16:213–7.

16. Reddy DN, Banerjee R, Choung OW. Antireflux biliary stents: are they the solution to stent occlusions? Curr Gastroenterol Rep 2006;8:156–60.

17. Dua KS, Reddy ND, Rao VG, et al. Impact of reducing duodenobiliary reflux on biliary stent patency: an in vitro evaluation and a prospective randomized clinical trial that used a biliary stent with an antireflux valve. Gastrointest Endosc 2007;65:819–28.

18. Raju GS, Sud R, Elfert AA, et al. Biliary drainage by using stents without a central lumen: a pilot study. Gastrointest Endosc 2006;63:317–20.

19. Kahaleh M, Tokar J, Le T, et al. Removal of self-expandable metallic Wallstents. Gastrointest Endosc 2004;60:640–4.

20. Deviere J, Cremer M, Baize M, et al. Management of common bile duct stricture caused by chronic pancreatitis with metal mesh self expandable stents. Gut 1994;35:122–6.
21. van Berkel AM, Cahen DL, van Westerloo DJ, et al. Self-expanding metal stents in benign biliary strictures due to chronic pancreatitis. Endoscopy 2004;36:381–4.
22. Kahaleh M, Behm B, Clarke BW, et al. Temporary placement of covered self-expandable metal stents in benign biliary strictures: a new paradigm? (with video). Gastrointest Endosc 2008;67:446–54.
23. Cantu P, Hookey LC, Morales A, et al. The treatment of patients with symptomatic common bile duct stenosis secondary to chronic pancreatitis using partially covered metal stents: a pilot study. Endoscopy 2005;37:735–9.
24. Bakhru MR, Kahaleh M. Expandable metal stents for benign biliary disease. Gastrointest Endosc Clin N Am 2011;21:447–62, viii.
25. Traina M, Tarantino I, Barresi L, et al. Efficacy and safety of fully covered self-expandable metallic stents in biliary complications after liver transplantation: a preliminary study. Liver Transpl 2009;15:1493–8.
26. Mahajan A, Ho H, Sauer B, et al. Temporary placement of fully covered self-expandable metal stents in benign biliary strictures: midterm evaluation (with video). Gastrointest Endosc 2009;70:303–9.
27. Chaput U, Scatton O, Bichard P, et al. Temporary placement of partially covered self-expandable metal stents for anastomotic biliary strictures after liver transplantation: a prospective, multicenter study. Gastrointest Endosc 2010;72:1167–74.
28. Kasher JA, Corasanti JG, Tarnasky PR, et al. A multicenter analysis of safety and outcome of removal of a fully covered self-expandable metal stent during ERCP. Gastrointest Endosc 2011;73:1292–7.
29. Phillips MS, Bonatti H, Sauer BG, et al. Elevated stricture rate following the use of fully covered self-expandable metal biliary stents for biliary leaks following liver transplantation. Endoscopy 2011;43:512–7.
30. Park do H, Lee SS, Lee TH, et al. Anchoring flap versus flared end, fully covered self-expandable metal stents to prevent migration in patients with benign biliary strictures: a multicenter, prospective, comparative pilot study (with videos). Gastrointest Endosc 2011;73:64–70.
31. Poley JW, van Tilburg AJ, Kuipers EJ, et al. Breaking the barrier: using extractable fully covered metal stents to treat benign biliary hilar strictures. Gastrointest Endosc 2011;74:916–20.
32. Park JK, Moon JH, Choi HJ, et al. Anchoring of a fully covered self-expandable metal stent with a 5F double-pigtail plastic stent to prevent migration in the management of benign biliary strictures. Am J Gastroenterol 2011;106:1761–5.
33. Thuluvath PJ, Pfau PR, Kimmey MB, et al. Biliary complications after liver transplantation: the role of endoscopy. Endoscopy 2005;37:857–63.
34. Smith MT, Sherman S, Lehman GA. Endoscopic management of benign strictures of the biliary tree. Endoscopy 1995;27:253–66.
35. Nimura Y, Kamiya J, Hayakawa N, et al. Cholangioscopic differentiation of biliary strictures and polyps. Endoscopy 1989;21(Suppl 1):351–6.
36. Kim HJ, Kim MH, Lee SK, et al. Tumor vessel: a valuable cholangioscopic clue of malignant biliary stricture. Gastrointest Endosc 2000;52:635–8.
37. Fukuda Y, Tsuyuguchi T, Sakai Y, et al. Diagnostic utility of peroral cholangioscopy for various bile-duct lesions. Gastrointest Endosc 2005;62:374–82.
38. Seo DW, Lee SK, Yoo KS, et al. Cholangioscopic findings in bile duct tumors. Gastrointest Endosc 2000;52:630–4.

39. Shah RJ, Langer DA, Antillon MR, et al. Cholangioscopy and cholangioscopic forceps biopsy in patients with indeterminate pancreaticobiliary pathology. Clin Gastroenterol Hepatol 2006;4:219–25.

40. Parsi MA, Guardino J, Vargo JJ. Peroral cholangioscopy-guided stricture therapy in living donor liver transplantation. Liver Transpl 2009;15:263–5.

41. Horwhat JD, Paulson EK, McGrath K, et al. A randomized comparison of EUS-guided FNA versus CT or US-guided FNA for the evaluation of pancreatic mass lesions. Gastrointest Endosc 2006;63:966–75.

42. Agarwal B, Abu-Hamda E, Molke KL, et al. Endoscopic ultrasound-guided fine needle aspiration and multidetector spiral CT in the diagnosis of pancreatic cancer. Am J Gastroenterol 2004;99:844–50.

43. Rosch T, Hofrichter K, Frimberger E, et al. ERCP or EUS for tissue diagnosis of biliary strictures? A prospective comparative study. Gastrointest Endosc 2004; 60:390–6.

44. Lee JH, Salem R, Aslanian H, et al. Endoscopic ultrasound and fine-needle aspiration of unexplained bile duct strictures. Am J Gastroenterol 2004;99:1069–73.

45. Garrow D, Miller S, Sinha D, et al. Endoscopic ultrasound: a meta-analysis of test performance in suspected biliary obstruction. Clin Gastroenterol Hepatol 2007;5:616–23.

46. Wu LM, Jiang XX, Gu HY, et al. Endoscopic ultrasound-guided fine-needle aspiration biopsy in the evaluation of bile duct strictures and gallbladder masses: a systematic review and meta-analysis. Eur J Gastroenterol Hepatol 2011;23: 113–20.

47. Kahaleh M, Hernandez AJ, Tokar J, et al. Interventional EUS-guided cholangiography: evaluation of a technique in evolution. Gastrointest Endosc 2006;64: 52–9.

48. Krishna NB, Saripalli S, Safdar R, et al. Intraductal US in evaluation of biliary strictures without a mass lesion on CT scan or magnetic resonance imaging: significance of focal wall thickening and extrinsic compression at the stricture site. Gastrointest Endosc 2007;66:90–6.

49. Iwashita T, Nakai Y, Lee JG, et al. A newly developed forward viewing echoendoscope - a comparative study to standard echoendoscope in imaging of abdominal organs and a feasibility of EUS-guided interventions. J Gastroenterol Hepatol 2012;27(2):362–7.

50. Vazquez-Sequeiros E, Baron TH, Clain JE, et al. Evaluation of indeterminate bile duct strictures by intraductal US. Gastrointest Endosc 2002;56:372–9.

51. Conway JD, Mishra G. The role of endoscopic ultrasound in biliary strictures. Curr Gastroenterol Rep 2008;10:157–62.

52. Meining A, Shah RJ, Slivka A, et al. Classification of probe-based confocal laser endomicroscopy findings in pancreaticobiliary strictures. Endoscopy 2012; 44(3):251–7.

53. Giovannini M, Bories E, Monges G, et al. Results of a phase I-II study on intraductal confocal microscopy (IDCM) in patients with common bile duct (CBD) stenosis. Surg Endosc 2011;25:2247–53.

54. Meining A, Chen YK, Pleskow D, et al. Direct visualization of indeterminate pancreaticobiliary strictures with probe-based confocal laser endomicroscopy: a multicenter experience. Gastrointest Endosc 2011;74:961–8.

55. Bergman JJ, van den Brink GR, Rauws EA, et al. Treatment of bile duct lesions after laparoscopic cholecystectomy. Gut 1996;38:141–7.

56. Lillemoe KD, Melton GB, Cameron JL, et al. Postoperative bile duct strictures: management and outcome in the 1990s. Ann Surg 2000;232:430–41.

57. Dolan JP, Diggs BS, Sheppard BC, et al. Ten-year trend in the national volume of bile duct injuries requiring operative repair. Surg Endosc 2005;19:967–73.
58. Peters JH, Ellison EC, Innes JT, et al. Safety and efficacy of laparoscopic cholecystectomy. A prospective analysis of 100 initial patients. Ann Surg 1991;213:3–12.
59. Costamagna G, Pandolfi M, Mutignani M, et al. Long-term results of endoscopic management of postoperative bile duct strictures with increasing numbers of stents. Gastrointest Endosc 2001;54:162–8.
60. Sicklick JK, Camp MS, Lillemoe KD, et al. Surgical management of bile duct injuries sustained during laparoscopic cholecystectomy: perioperative results in 200 patients. Ann Surg 2005;241:786–92 [discussion: 93–5].
61. Sikora SS, Pottakkal B, Srikanth G, et al. Postcholecystectomy benign biliary strictures - long-term results. Dig Surg 2006;23:304–12.
62. Bergman JJ, Burgemeister L, Bruno MJ, et al. Long-term follow-up after biliary stent placement for postoperative bile duct stenosis. Gastrointest Endosc 2001; 54:154–61.
63. Davids PH, Rauws EA, Coene PP, et al. Endoscopic stenting for post-operative biliary strictures. Gastrointest Endosc 1992;38:12–8.
64. Weber A, Feussner H, Winkelmann F, et al. Long-term outcome of endoscopic therapy in patients with bile duct injury after cholecystectomy. J Gastroenterol Hepatol 2009;24:762–9.
65. Draganov P, Hoffman B, Marsh W, et al. Long-term outcome in patients with benign biliary strictures treated endoscopically with multiple stents. Gastrointest Endosc 2002;55:680–6.
66. Kassab C, Prat F, Liguory C, et al. Endoscopic management of post-laparoscopic cholecystectomy biliary strictures. Long-term outcome in a multi-center study. Gastroenterol Clin Biol 2006;30:124–9.
67. Greif F, Bronsther OL, Van Thiel DH, et al. The incidence, timing, and management of biliary tract complications after orthotopic liver transplantation. Ann Surg 1994;219:40–5.
68. Park JS, Kim MH, Lee SK, et al. Efficacy of endoscopic and percutaneous treatments for biliary complications after cadaveric and living donor liver transplantation. Gastrointest Endosc 2003;57:78–85.
69. Thethy S, Thomson B, Pleass H, et al. Management of biliary tract complications after orthotopic liver transplantation. Clin Transplant 2004;18:647–53.
70. Gunawansa N, McCall JL, Holden A, et al. Biliary complications following orthotopic liver transplantation: a 10-year audit. HPB (Oxford) 2011;13:391–9.
71. Gondolesi GE, Varotti G, Florman SS, et al. Biliary complications in 96 consecutive right lobe living donor transplant recipients. Transplantation 2004;77: 1842–8.
72. Todo S, Furukawa H, Kamiyama T. How to prevent and manage biliary complications in living donor liver transplantation? J Hepatol 2005;43:22–7.
73. Pascher A, Neuhaus P. Biliary complications after deceased-donor orthotopic liver transplantation. J Hepatobiliary Pancreat Surg 2006;13:487–96.
74. Testa G, Malago M, Broelseh CE. Complications of biliary tract in liver transplantation. World J Surg 2001;25:1296–9.
75. Welling TH, Heidt DG, Englesbe MJ, et al. Biliary complications following liver transplantation in the model for end-stage liver disease era: effect of donor, recipient, and technical factors. Liver Transpl 2008;14:73–80.
76. Foley DP, Fernandez LA, Leverson G, et al. Donation after cardiac death: the University of Wisconsin experience with liver transplantation. Ann Surg 2005; 242:724–31.

77. Tsujino T, Isayama H, Sugawara Y, et al. Endoscopic management of biliary complications after adult living donor liver transplantation. Am J Gastroenterol 2006;101:2230–6.
78. Shah JN, Ahmad NA, Shetty K, et al. Endoscopic management of biliary complications after adult living donor liver transplantation. Am J Gastroenterol 2004;99: 1291–5.
79. Londono MC, Balderramo D, Cardenas A. Management of biliary complications after orthotopic liver transplantation: the role of endoscopy. World J Gastroenterol 2008;14:493–7.
80. Hussaini SH, Sheridan MB, Davies M. The predictive value of transabdominal ultrasonography in the diagnosis of biliary tract complications after orthotopic liver transplantation. Gut 1999;45:900–3.
81. Linhares MM, Gonzalez AM, Goldman SM, et al. Magnetic resonance cholangiography in the diagnosis of biliary complications after orthotopic liver transplantation. Transplant Proc 2004;36:947–8.
82. Fulcher AS, Turner MA. Orthotopic liver transplantation: evaluation with MR cholangiography. Radiology 1999;211:715–22.
83. Kurzawinski TR, Selves L, Farouk M, et al. Prospective study of hepatobiliary scintigraphy and endoscopic cholangiography for the detection of early biliary complications after orthotopic liver transplantation. Br J Surg 1997;84:620–3.
84. Lerut J, Gordon RD, Iwatsuki S, et al. Biliary tract complications in human orthotopic liver transplantation. Transplantation 1987;43:47–51.
85. Ito K, Siegelman ES, Stolpen AH, et al. MR imaging of complications after liver transplantation. AJR Am J Roentgenol 2000;175:1145–9.
86. Graziadei IW, Schwaighofer H, Koch R, et al. Long-term outcome of endoscopic treatment of biliary strictures after liver transplantation. Liver Transpl 2006;12: 718–25.
87. Guichelaar MM, Benson JT, Malinchoc M, et al. Risk factors for and clinical course of non-anastomotic biliary strictures after liver transplantation. Am J Transplant 2003;3:885–90.
88. Pasha SF, Harrison ME, Das A, et al. Endoscopic treatment of anastomotic biliary strictures after deceased donor liver transplantation: outcomes after maximal stent therapy. Gastrointest Endosc 2007;66:44–51.
89. Verdonk RC, Buis CI, van der Jagt EJ, et al. Nonanastomotic biliary strictures after liver transplantation, part 2: management, outcome, and risk factors for disease progression. Liver Transpl 2007;13:725–32.
90. Schwartz DA, Petersen BT, Poterucha JJ, et al. Endoscopic therapy of anastomotic bile duct strictures occurring after liver transplantation. Gastrointest Endosc 2000;51:169–74.
91. Zoepf T, Maldonado-Lopez EJ, Hilgard P, et al. Balloon dilatation vs. balloon dilatation plus bile duct endoprostheses for treatment of anastomotic biliary strictures after liver transplantation. Liver Transpl 2006;12:88–94.
92. Morelli J, Mulcahy HE, Willner IR, et al. Long-term outcomes for patients with post-liver transplant anastomotic biliary strictures treated by endoscopic stent placement. Gastrointest Endosc 2003;58:374–9.
93. Kulaksiz H, Weiss KH, Gotthardt D, et al. Is stenting necessary after balloon dilation of post-transplantation biliary strictures? Results of a prospective comparative study. Endoscopy 2008;40:746–51.
94. Garcia-Pajares F, Sanchez-Antolin G, Pelayo SL, et al. Covered metal stents for the treatment of biliary complications after orthotopic liver transplantation. Transplant Proc 2010;42:2966–9.

95. Hu B, Gao DJ, Yu FH, et al. Endoscopic stenting for post-transplant biliary stricture: usefulness of a novel removable covered metal stent. J Hepatobiliary Pancreat Sci 2011;18:640–5.

96. Tee HP, James MW, Kaffes AJ. Placement of removable metal biliary stent in post-orthotopic liver transplantation anastomotic stricture. World J Gastroenterol 2010;16:3597–600.

97. Tada S, Yazumi S, Chiba T. Endoscopic management is an accepted first-line therapy for biliary complications after adult living donor liver transplantation. Am J Gastroenterol 2007;102:1331 [author reply: 2].

98. Rizk RS, McVicar JP, Emond MJ, et al. Endoscopic management of biliary strictures in liver transplant recipients: effect on patient and graft survival. Gastrointest Endosc 1998;47:128–35.

99. Stahl TJ, Allen MO, Ansel HJ, et al. Partial biliary obstruction caused by chronic pancreatitis. An appraisal of indications for surgical biliary drainage. Ann Surg 1988;207:26–32.

100. Aranha GV, Prinz RA, Freeark RJ, et al. The spectrum of biliary tract obstruction from chronic pancreatitis. Arch Surg 1984;119:595–600.

101. Hammel P, Couvelard A, O'Toole D, et al. Regression of liver fibrosis after biliary drainage in patients with chronic pancreatitis and stenosis of the common bile duct. N Engl J Med 2001;344:418–23.

102. Kiehne K, Folsch UR, Nitsche R. High complication rate of bile duct stents in patients with chronic alcoholic pancreatitis due to noncompliance. Endoscopy 2000;32:377–80.

103. Cahen DL, van Berkel AM, Oskam D, et al. Long-term results of endoscopic drainage of common bile duct strictures in chronic pancreatitis. Eur J Gastroenterol Hepatol 2005;17:103–8.

104. Pozsar J, Sahin P, Laszlo F, et al. Medium-term results of endoscopic treatment of common bile duct strictures in chronic calcifying pancreatitis with increasing numbers of stents. J Clin Gastroenterol 2004;38:118–23.

105. Yamaguchi T, Ishihara T, Seza K, et al. Long-term outcome of endoscopic metallic stenting for benign biliary stenosis associated with chronic pancreatitis. World J Gastroenterol 2006;12:426–30.

106. Sauer BG, Regan KA, Srinivasan I. 347e: Temporary placement of covered self-expandable metal stents (CSEMS) in benign biliary strictures (BBS): eight years of experience. Gastrointest Endosc 2010;71:AB110–1.

107. MacCarty RL, LaRusso NF, Wiesner RH, et al. Primary sclerosing cholangitis: findings on cholangiography and pancreatography. Radiology 1983;149:39–44.

108. Tischendorf JJ, Hecker H, Kruger M, et al. Characterization, outcome, and prognosis in 273 patients with primary sclerosing cholangitis: a single center study. Am J Gastroenterol 2007;102:107–14.

109. Stiehl A, Rudolph G, Kloters-Plachky P, et al. Development of dominant bile duct stenoses in patients with primary sclerosing cholangitis treated with ursodeoxycholic acid: outcome after endoscopic treatment. J Hepatol 2002;36:151–6.

110. Okolicsanyi L, Fabris L, Viaggi S, et al. Primary sclerosing cholangitis: clinical presentation, natural history and prognostic variables: an Italian multicentre study. The Italian PSC Study Group. Eur J Gastroenterol Hepatol 1996;8:685–91.

111. Tischendorf JJ, Kruger M, Trautwein C, et al. Cholangioscopic characterization of dominant bile duct stenoses in patients with primary sclerosing cholangitis. Endoscopy 2006;38:665–9.

112. Farrant JM, Hayllar KM, Wilkinson ML, et al. Natural history and prognostic variables in primary sclerosing cholangitis. Gastroenterology 1991;100: 1710–7.

113. Beuers U, Spengler U, Kruis W, et al. Ursodeoxycholic acid for treatment of primary sclerosing cholangitis: a placebo-controlled trial. Hepatology 1992;16: 707–14.

114. Levy MJ, Baron TH, Clayton AC, et al. Prospective evaluation of advanced molecular markers and imaging techniques in patients with indeterminate bile duct strictures. Am J Gastroenterol 2008;103:1263–73.

115. Petersen-Benz C, Stiehl A. Impact of dominant stenoses on the serum level of the tumor marker CA19-9 in patients with primary sclerosing cholangitis. Z Gastroenterol 2005;43:587–90.

116. Ponsioen CY, Vrouenraets SM, van Milligen de Wit AW, et al. Value of brush cytology for dominant strictures in primary sclerosing cholangitis. Endoscopy 1999;31:305–9.

117. Barr Fritcher EG, Kipp BR, Voss JS, et al. Primary sclerosing cholangitis patients with serial polysomy fluorescence in situ hybridization results are at increased risk of cholangiocarcinoma. Am J Gastroenterol 2011;106:2023–8.

118. Weber C, Kuhlencordt R, Grotelueschen R, et al. Magnetic resonance cholangiopancreatography in the diagnosis of primary sclerosing cholangitis. Endoscopy 2008;40:739–45.

119. Moff SL, Kamel IR, Eustace J, et al. Diagnosis of primary sclerosing cholangitis: a blinded comparative study using magnetic resonance cholangiography and endoscopic retrograde cholangiography. Gastrointest Endosc 2006;64: 219–23.

120. Bangarulingam SY, Gossard AA, Petersen BT, et al. Complications of endoscopic retrograde cholangiopancreatography in primary sclerosing cholangitis. Am J Gastroenterol 2009;104:855–60.

121. van Milligen de Wit AW, van Bracht J, Rauws EA, et al. Endoscopic stent therapy for dominant extrahepatic bile duct strictures in primary sclerosing cholangitis. Gastrointest Endosc 1996;44:293–9.

122. Lee JG, Schutz SM, England RE, et al. Endoscopic therapy of sclerosing cholangitis. Hepatology 1995;21:661–7.

123. Stiehl A, Rudolph G, Sauer P, et al. Efficacy of ursodeoxycholic acid treatment and endoscopic dilation of major duct stenoses in primary sclerosing cholangitis. An 8-year prospective study. J Hepatol 1997;26:560–6.

124. Baluyut AR, Sherman S, Lehman GA, et al. Impact of endoscopic therapy on the survival of patients with primary sclerosing cholangitis. Gastrointest Endosc 2001;53:308–12.

125. Gluck M, Cantone NR, Brandabur JJ, et al. A twenty-year experience with endoscopic therapy for symptomatic primary sclerosing cholangitis. J Clin Gastroenterol 2008;42:1032–9.

126. Kaya M, Petersen BT, Angulo P, et al. Balloon dilation compared to stenting of dominant strictures in primary sclerosing cholangitis. Am J Gastroenterol 2001;96:1059–66.

127. Ponsioen CY, Lam K, van Milligen de Wit AW, et al. Four years experience with short term stenting in primary sclerosing cholangitis. Am J Gastroenterol 1999; 94:2403–7.

128. Nakazawa T, Ohara H, Sano H, et al. Cholangiography can discriminate sclerosing cholangitis with autoimmune pancreatitis from primary sclerosing cholangitis. Gastrointest Endosc 2004;60:937–44.

129. Nakazawa T, Naitoh I, Hayashi K, et al. Diagnostic criteria for IgG4-related sclerosing cholangitis based on cholangiographic classification. J Gastroenterol 2012;47(1):79–87.
130. Kalaitzakis E, Levy M, Kamisawa T, et al. Endoscopic retrograde cholangiography does not reliably distinguish IgG4-associated cholangitis from primary sclerosing cholangitis or cholangiocarcinoma. Clin Gastroenterol Hepatol 2011;9:800–3 e2.
131. Benhamou Y, Caumes E, Gerosa Y, et al. AIDS-related cholangiopathy. Critical analysis of a prospective series of 26 patients. Dig Dis Sci 1993;38:1113–8.
132. Cello JP, Chan MF. Long-term follow-up of endoscopic retrograde cholangiopancreatography sphincterotomy for patients with acquired immune deficiency syndrome papillary stenosis. Am J Med 1995;99:600–3.
133. Castiella A, Iribarren JA, Lopez P, et al. Ursodeoxycholic acid in the treatment of AIDS-associated cholangiopathy. Am J Med 1997;103:170–1.
134. Bayraktar Y. Portal ductopathy: clinical importance and nomenclature. World J Gastroenterol 2011;17:1410–5.
135. Dilawari JB, Chawla YK. Pseudosclerosing cholangitis in extrahepatic portal venous obstruction. Gut 1992;33:272–6.
136. Khuroo MS, Yattoo GN, Zargar SA, et al. Biliary abnormalities associated with extrahepatic portal venous obstruction. Hepatology 1993;17:807–13.
137. Dhiman RK, Puri P, Chawla Y, et al. Biliary changes in extrahepatic portal venous obstruction: compression by collaterals or ischemic? Gastrointest Endosc 1999; 50:646–52.
138. Saleem A, Baron TH, Gostout CJ, et al. Endoscopic retrograde cholangiopancreatography using a single-balloon enteroscope in patients with altered Roux-en-Y anatomy. Endoscopy 2010;42:656–60.
139. Wang AY, Sauer BG, Behm BW, et al. Single-balloon enteroscopy effectively enables diagnostic and therapeutic retrograde cholangiography in patients with surgically altered anatomy. Gastrointest Endosc 2010;71:641–9.
140. Bruno M, Boermeester M, Rauws E, et al. Use of removable covered expandable metal stents (RCEMS) in the treatment of benign distal common bile duct (CBD) strictures: a feasibility study. Gastrointest Endosc 2005;61:AB199.
141. Tringali A, Di Matteo F, Iacopini F, et al. Common bile duct strictures due to chronic pancreatitis managed by self-expandable-metal stents (SEMS): results of a long-term follow-up study. Gastrointest Endosc 2005;61:AB220.
142. Kuo MD, Lopresti DC, Gover DD, et al. Intentional retrieval of Viabil stent-grafts from the biliary system. J Vasc Interv Radiol 2006;17:389–97.
143. Cahen DL, Rauws EA, Gouma DJ, et al. Removable fully covered self-expandable metal stents in the treatment of common bile duct strictures due to chronic pancreatitis: a case series. Endoscopy 2008;40:697–700.

Treatment of Common Bile Duct Injuries After Surgery

Claudio Navarrete, MD, Jaquelina M. Gobelet, MD*

KEYWORDS

- Bile duct injuries • Bile fistula • Biliary stenosis • Liver transplantation
- Self-expandable stent • Endoscopic management

KEY POINTS

- The treatment of common biliary duct injuries after surgery remains a challenge for physicians.
- The management of biliary tract injuries will depend on the nature and extent of the injury, the presence or absence of biloma, and time to diagnosis of the injury. It should be performed in referral centers.
- The lesions of the bile ducts are divided into fistulas and stenosis.
- In biliary fistulas, the goal of endoscopic therapy is to reduce the pressure of the sphincter of Oddi with nasobiliary drainage, biliary sphincterotomy, or placement of prosthesis with or without sphincterotomy.
- For biliary strictures the objectives are to relieve the obstruction, prevent restenosis, and prevent hepatocellular damage.
- The treatment of biliary injuries after surgery needs a multidisciplinary team.

Endoscopic treatment of bile duct injury is a permanent challenge for endoscopists, and endoscopic retrograde cholangiopancreatography (ERCP) is a valuable tool in this field.

This article discusses the endoscopic management of biliary fistulas and postsurgical stenosis including liver transplantation. It also aims to provide tools to determine when and how endoscopic management may be the treatment of choice in a patient with a surgical complication of the biliary tract. Practical information on the management of these complications is also given.

CLASSIFICATION

There are multiple classifications, of which the Strasberg classification remains the most widespread and widely used. Strasberg classifies the biliary tract injuries according to

The authors have nothing to disclose.
The Latin American Gastrointestinal Endoscopy Training Center, Endoscopy Division, Clinica Alemana Santiago, Universidad del Desarrollo, Santiago de Chile 7630000, Chile
* Corresponding author.
E-mail address: jaquigobelet@yahoo.com.ar

Gastrointest Endoscopy Clin N Am 22 (2012) 539–553
doi:10.1016/j.giec.2012.04.023
1052-5157/12/$ – see front matter © 2012 Elsevier Inc. All rights reserved.

giendo.theclinics.com

anatomic considerations and therapeutic alternatives. The authors recommend Strasberg because it identifies potential endoscopically treatable lesions and also because it is widely accepted by surgical teams (**Fig. 1**).[1]

There are no management algorithms based on evidence that allow determination of which lesions of the biliary tract improve with ERCP. At present the indications and contraindications for endoscopic management are based primarily on recommendations from experts, supported by facts such as the extent of the injury, fistula flow, the time when the lesion is diagnosed in the intraoperative or postoperative period, the presence of sterile or infected biloma, and the risk associated with surgical repair (**Table 1**).[2]

ENDOSCOPIC MANAGEMENT CONSIDERATIONS
Nature and Extent of Injury

The presence of continuity of the bile duct is the most important factor in determining the ability to manage the injury by endoscopy. If there is continuity of the bile duct (lesion types Strasberg A, C, and D), ERCP is considered the primary therapy. On the other hand, the endoscopic management is often not possible in the presence of injuries that completely transect the bile duct, when there are clips on the distal stump and when there is no continuity between the injured segments (injury types Strasberg B or E).[3,4]

Although the authors have successfully treated complete transection of the bile duct by ERCP, without requiring a simultaneous transhepatic percutaneous access, these cases should be considered anecdotal. Complete transection of the bile duct is a strong indication for surgery. Exclusive use of endoscopic treatment is to be considered only if one can successfully cross the lesion and completely decompress the bile duct using prosthesis.

Aberrant bile ducts usually drain bile from liver segments directly to the gallbladder bed or common bile duct, and rarely to the right or left bile duct. If an inadvertent injury of an aberrant duct occurs during surgery, an ERCP is likely to be required. If the contrast displays an aberrant duct, this means that the latter is connected to the biliary tract, so ERCP would be therapeutic if a sphincterotomy is performed, a biliary stent placed, and/or cyanoacrylate is injected. If the injury is not visible during ERCP, other studies such as scintigraphy or cholangioresonance will be required, and the resolution will likely be surgical resection.[5]

Flow Through the Fistula

A clinically significant biliary fistula is a potentially serious complication that is reported in 0.1% to 0.5% of classic cholecystectomies and goes up to 2% in cases of laparoscopic cholecystectomies.

The cystic duct is the most common leak site (78%), followed by an aberrant right hepatic duct of Luschka (13%) and other sites (9%) such as the common hepatic bile duct and the point of insertion of the Kehr tube. High-flow fistulas were traditionally considered for surgical resolution, but there are now several reports of successful endoscopic treatment (**Table 2**).

Shanda and colleagues[6] defined the low-flow fistula as one that appears only after contrasting the intrahepatic bile duct and the high-flow fistula as one that is recognized before contrasting the intrahepatic bile duct. ERCP is generally used as a diagnostic method in suspected biliary fistula, and endoscopic management should be attempted even in the case of a high-flow fistula.

The most common biliary fistulas originate within the cystic duct, either by failure of the clip, drop of the clip, or thermal injury of the cystic remnant. Injury to the Luschka

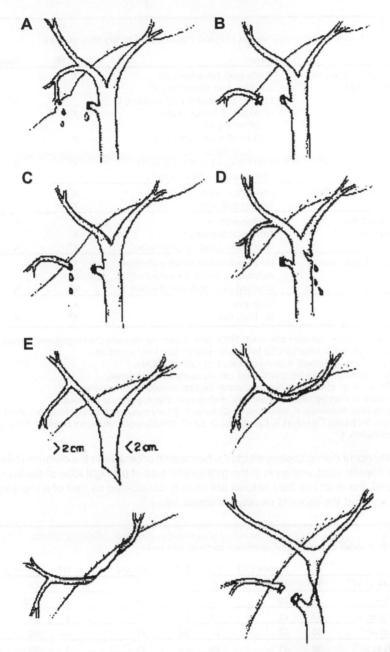

Fig. 1. Classification of biliary injury during laparoscopic cholecystectomy. Type A is a transection of small bile ducts that are entered in the liver bed or from the cystic duct. Types B and C almost always involve aberrant right hepatic ducts. Type D is a tear or burn of the common bile duct (CBD). Type E implies transection or resection of the CBD. Type A, C, D, and some E injuries frequently cause bilomas of fistulas, requiring external drainage. Type B is considered as initially treated. (*Adapted from* Strasberg SM, Hertl M, Soper NJ. An analysis of the problem of biliary injury during laparoscopic cholecystectomy. J Am Coll Surg 1995;180(1):101–25; with permission.)

Table 1
Factors influencing endoscopic versus surgical treatment of biliary tree injuries

	Factor	ECRP	Surgery
Nature and magnitude of the lesion	Cystic duct (Strasberg A)	X	
	Luschka duct (Strasberg A)	X	
	Ligated sectorial duct (Strasberg B)		X[a]
	Nonligated sectorial duct (Strasberg C)	X[b]	X
	CBD small tearing/burning (Strasberg D)	X	
	CBD transection (Strasberg E)	X[c]	X
	CBD resection (Strasberg E)		X
Flow through the leak	Low-grade leak	X	
	High-grade leak	X[d]	X
Time to set the diagnosis	Intraoperative		X
	Early postoperative	X	
	Late postoperative (strictures)	X[d]	X
Associated collections	No associated or small collection	X	
	Aseptic, no septated collection	X	
	Infected or septated collection	X[e]	X
Surgical risk	High risk	X	
	No high risk	X[d]	X

Abbreviations: CBD, common bile duct; ERCP, endoscopic retrograde cholangiopancreatography.
[a] Absent communication to CBD branches lead to late liver resection.
[b] Only if aberrant system is communicated to CBD branches.
[c] Only if continuity can be established can stenting be considered.
[d] ERCP seems as effective as surgery; other factors should be considered.
[e] Drainage is priority; after completion, endoscopic therapy should be used.
Adapted from Navarrete C, Valdivieso E, Gobelet J. Biliary surgery complications including transplantation. In: Baron T, Kosarek R, Carr-Locke D. ERCP. Philadelphia: Saunders Elsevier; 2008. p. 338; with permission.

duct may occur during cholecystectomy because it originates in the common bile duct or right hepatic duct, and ends in the gallbladder bed of the right lobe of the liver.

Instead, the main bile duct fistulas are usually considered as part of a more extensive injury, and the cause is usually a thermal injury.[2]

Table 2
Published series of endoscopic approach to treat bile leaks

Series	n	Stones (%)	ES	Stent	ES and Stent	NT	Efficacy (%)
Kozarek et al[20]	11	18	2	7	—	1	82
Foutch et al[19]	23	30	4	6	12	1	100
Barkum et al[10]	52	22	27	1	27	8	88
Ryan et al[23]	50	22	6	13	31	—	88
Davids et al[18]	48	31	20	—	25	3	90
Prat et al[51]	26	31	15	—	3	8	70
De Palma et al[21]	64	33	25	18	—	21	96.9
Sandha et al[6]	204	20	75	—	—	—	99

Abbreviations: ES, endoscopic sphincterotomy; NT, nasobiliary tube.
Adapted from Navarrete C, Valdivieso E, Gobelet J. Biliary surgery complications including transplantation. In: Baron T, Kosarek R, Carr-Locke D. ERCP. Philadelphia: Saunders Elsevier; 2008. p. 338; with permission.

Time to Diagnosis

If a patient is diagnosed with a bile duct injury in the postoperative period (early or late), the treatment of choice is endoscopic. If the injury is diagnosed intraoperatively, it should be resolved during the same surgical procedure. However, a stent may be used to ensure biliary drainage after a choledochorrhaphy.[7]

Management of the Lesions of the Biliary Tract

As already mentioned, the management of biliary tract injuries will depend on the nature and extent of the injury, the presence or absence of biloma, and time to diagnosis of the injury. Most injuries are recognized in the period after cholecystectomy, and only 25% to 36% are recognized during laparoscopic cholecystectomy.[8]

It is important to make a thorough evaluation of the patient to ensure early recognition of injury and prevent a deterioration that might end in peritonitis, sepsis, or even death.

Successful treatment of these complications requires a multidisciplinary group that includes biliary endoscopists, interventional radiologists, and hepatobiliary surgeons. It is important to refer patients to tertiary centers with experience in the management of these lesions, which has been proved to reduce related morbidity and mortality rates.[9]

To address this issue, according to the Strasberg classification the authors divided the lesions of the bile ducts into those presenting fistulas and those for which the main manifestation is biliary stenosis.

BILIARY FISTULA

Small biliary fistulas are common after cholecystectomy. If postoperative ultrasonography was performed routinely, small fluid collections would be detected in the gallbladder bed in 24% of patients. Most of these resolve spontaneously, without requiring any procedure.[8] By contrast, approximately 0.8% to 1.1% of patients had significant postoperative biliary fistulas that were suspected as being due to persistent biliary drainage through the T-tube or drainage tubes, or symptoms of pain and fever associated with distension, ileus, and jaundice.[10,11] This condition usually occurs during the first postoperative week but sometimes can take up to 30 days. The diagnosis is confirmed by abdominal ultrasonography, computed tomography, or cholangiography through T-tube.[12] Endoscopic cholangiography plays an important role in determining the site of the biliary fistula. In about 95% of patients the site of the fistula is diagnosed through the loss of contrast during cholangiography (**Fig. 2**). Its high sensitivity makes cholangiography nowadays the radiologic method of choice, also allowing a therapeutic intervention.[13]

The goal of endoscopic therapy is to reduce the pressure of the sphincter of Oddi, allowing transpapillary bile flow and avoiding extravasation in the fistula site. The type of treatment chosen by the endoscopist will depend on the size of the fistula, the presence of biloma, and whether there is presence of residual bile duct calculus.[14,15]

Endoscopic therapy is empiric, and a systematic approach in relation to the size of the fistula has not been established. The alternatives include nasobiliary drainage, biliary sphincterotomy alone, placement of prosthesis with or without sphincterotomy, and in the presence of a residual calculus, its removal. Nasobiliary drainage has the advantage of being installed without the need for a sphincterotomy and allows repeated cholangiograms without the need for new endoscopic procedures. Although used in some centers, in the authors' practice nasobiliary drainage is rarely used

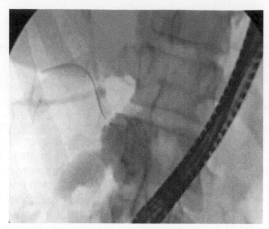

Fig. 2. Biliary leak. Strasberg A.

because of the discomfort caused to the patient and the risk of accidental or deliberate removal.[6,16]

Biliary sphincterotomy and installation of a biliary stent are widely used and are considered successful techniques in most cases. Although there are no randomized studies comparing different techniques, there are several series that evaluate different endoscopic approaches and report a success rate of 88% to 100%, although the overall results are difficult to compare because the choice of therapies was not based on the severity of the fistula.[10,17–22]

A North American multicenter study evaluated the efficacy of different endoscopic therapies in 50 patients and showed comparable efficacy to previous series with a follow-up of 17.5 months. The most frequently used was the therapeutic sphincterotomy with placement of a 7F or 10F stent for 4 to 6 weeks (62%). Bile fistulas were classified as high grade or low grade; however, this classification was not used to determine the endoscopic approach.[23]

In a Canadian study, Sandha and colleagues[6] proposed systematic endoscopic therapy for the treatment of biliary fistulas based on the severity of the bile leak in 207 patients referred within 9 days postoperatively. The most common sites affected were the cystic duct and Luschka duct. Sphincterotomy alone was empirically used for low-grade fistulas, and the prosthesis, with or without sphincterotomy, for 4 to 6 weeks for high-grade fistulas. Ninety-one percent of patients with low-grade fistulas and 97% with high-grade fistulas resolved. The complication rate was 1.5% (2 pancreatitis, 1 perforation). Even though this is not a randomized controlled trial, the different endoscopic therapies were applied consistently and the results confirm the value of a simple classification system.

In 20% to 25% of cases residual bile duct calculus can be detected. If the fistula is low grade, biliary sphincterotomy with stone removal alone is sufficient in most cases, but if the fistula is high grade it is also preferable to place a biliary stent, because sphincterotomy does not always completely eliminate the gradient transpapillary pressure.[6]

Considering that a sphincterotomy does not always section the whole sphincter, the authors recommend performing a sphincterotomy plus installation of a 4-to 5-cm 7F prosthetic stent, thus reducing the risk of perforation and bleeding from a wide sphincterotomy.[24]

There are no studies comparing the number and size of the stent to be installed, nor is there much clarity with respect to time to be left in situ. In their center the authors usually place one 7F prosthesis when the fistula is in the cystic duct or in the Luschka accessory bile duct without evidence of stenosis; the patient is then followed up for 4 weeks and if there is no leak, the prosthesis is removed. In the event of any major damage to the bile duct or when a stenosis is suspected, the authors prefer to install a 10F prosthesis and the largest amount possible, complying with the management of bile duct stenosis, as detailed in the following section.[25]

The benefits of a self-expandable prosthesis are widely known in the palliative management of malignant diseases, but in recent times their usefulness in benign conditions has begun to be explored. In complex biliary fistulas, which do not respond to a plastic stent and sphincterotomy, the use of a fully covered self-expandable prosthesis not only reduces the pressure of the sphincter of Oddi but may also close the fistula area. Because these stents are fully covered, their subsequent removal is facilitated and additionally they do not damage the bile duct, preventing subsequent stricture formation. Although there are some studies with promising results and low complication rates, randomized trials comparing plastic prostheses with self-expandable ones are required before making a firm recommendation regarding their use.[26]

Twenty-five percent of patients also require percutaneous drainage of collections. Bilomas that extends outside the gallbladder bed or those that are larger than 3 cm should be drained percutaneously, with only a small percentage requiring surgical drainage (4%–6%).[23]

Recommendation

Endoscopic treatment is the therapy of choice for postcholecystectomy biliary fistulas as shown by most published series, with a success rate of more than 90%.

STENOSIS OF BILIARY DUCT

Benign strictures of the biliary tree remain a challenge. Although important technological development has led to improved diagnostic and therapeutic methodology, the high morbidity and mortality associated with this entity represent a serious clinical problem.

The objective in the management of biliary strictures is to relieve obstruction, and prevent restenosis and secondary hepatocellular damage. Duct injuries are recognized intraoperatively in about 25% of patients, and many can be repaired inmediately.[11] For patients in whom the injury is not recognized, the nature and time of clinical presentation is variable and depends on the type of injury. The coexistence of a biliary fistula leads to an earlier presentation of symptoms, as outlined in the previous section.

By contrast, in those who develop stenosis without fistula, symptoms may appear weeks or months later with signs of biliary obstruction such as jaundice, cholestasis in the laboratory, and biliary dilatation on ultrasonography. These patients have Strasberg E-type injuries.

The location of the stenosis is very important not only for therapeutic management but also for establishing prognosis (**Fig. 3**). Thus, Strasberg E1 and E2 lesions offer the best prognosis.[27]

Early diagnosis is, therefore, imperative and early images are needed. Ultrasonography and computed axial tomography can detect biliary dilatation or collections. Magnetic resonance cholangiography allows imaging of the biliary tree and location of the site of stenosis. Although helpful for further treatment, not being a dynamic radiologic study it does not allow differentiation of biliary stenosis from complete biliary transection. Transhepatic cholangiography or ERCP, in addition to defining the anatomy of

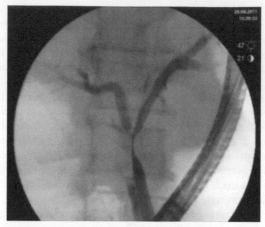

Fig. 3. Postcholecystectomy confluence stenosis. Strasberg E3.

the biliary tract and identifying the site of the stenosis, allow their treatment. Magnetic resonance cholangiography may be preferred in patients with complete biliary disconnection that excludes the use of ERCP, but it does not determine which patient suffers from a biliary duct disconnection until a dynamic contrast study is performed.

There is still controversy about the optimal treatment algorithm for these patients. Strictures of the bile duct have traditionally been the territory of surgeons, leaving a limited role to endoscopy. There are no prospective controlled studies comparing surgery with endoscopy, perhaps because of the relative infrequency of this problem and the heterogeneity of the lesions.[28–30]

It is important that when evaluating the results of different techniques, optimization of surgical outcomes is best achieved through the management of these complications by surgeons experienced in bile duct treatment (**Fig. 4**).

In a retrospective report published by Davids and colleagues[30] in 1993, the results of endoscopic therapy versus surgery were compared. Thirty-five patients in the surgery group and 66 in the endoscopic group with comparable biliary injury were analyzed. During the endoscopic treatment, cholangitis occurred in 21% of cases but all responded to the change of prosthesis. In the surgical group, 17% developed recurrent stenosis requiring further surgery. Follow-up was 4 years, and a success rate comparable in both groups of around 83% was obtained.

The factors influencing the results are primarily the level of stenosis and the type of stenosis, and patients with Strasberg E3, E4 or E5 have a lower success rate compared with those with Strasberg E1 and E2, independent of whether the treatment is endoscopic or surgical.[27,30–32] The patients having a segment disconnection or complete transection injury should, by definition, undergo surgical management. In these cases endoscopic therapy is not recommended.

In a series of retrospective studies that evaluated the surgical management of post-laparoscopy bile duct lesions (resection and hepaticojejunal anastomosis), high rates of improvement were shown with this technique, although the best results were obtained in those patients with a higher percentage of Strasberg E1 and E2 stenosis.[33–35]

A prospective study including 142 patients showed a long-term success rate of 98% with surgery after insertion of a biliary stent.[36]

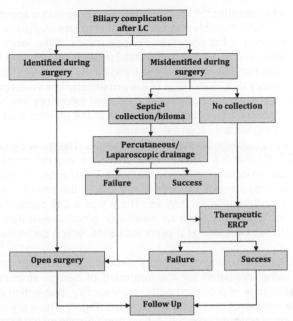

Fig. 4. ERCP for treatment of complications after laparoscopic cholecystectomy. [a]In selected cases of septic collections and/or biloma, open surgery could be indicated as primary treatment. (*Adapted from* Navarrete C, Valdivieso E, Gobelet J. Biliary surgery complications including transplantation. In: Baron T, Kosarek R, Carr-Locke D. ERCP. Philadelphia: Saunders Elsevier; 2008. p. 339; with permission.)

Other important factors are the type of surgery performed in the first approach, the surgical center, and the time of diagnosis. The patients who initially underwent reconstructive repair in experienced centers showed lower restenosis rates than those patients with previous reparative attempts who were referred to tertiary centers in a late phase (2.5%–25%). In addition, the surgical failure rate is higher in primary centers than in more experienced centers (83% vs 6%).[27]

Reconstructive surgery performed during the early postoperative period was associated with a higher complication rate compared with that made 2 or 3 months later (80% vs 17%), probably because of local inflammatory reaction that accompanies the surgery.[11]

In attempts at a less invasive approach for these patients, different endoscopic techniques have been proposed as an alternative to hepaticojejunal anastomosis, including balloon dilatation and stent placement, and although many differences between the techniques have not been clearly established, good results comparable with surgery have been shown.[29]

Most studies report good results with the double insertion of a 10F prosthesis for a year with refills every 3 to 4 months.

When balloon dilatation is used as monotherapy it is not a successful technique because its long-term effect is not permanent, but it is useful in facilitating the installation of a prosthesis.[37]

One of the largest series[38] included 74 patients with long-term follow-up of 9 years. The success rate was 80% and restenosis was observed in 20% of cases, with a mortality related to procedure of 2% to 3%.

Costamagna and colleagues[39,40] proposed a more aggressive approach, insertion of stents on the maximum possible number in relation to size and diameter of stenosis of the bile duct, to achieve the complete disappearance of the lesion. The average number of prostheses was 1 to 4 during the initial session and 1 to 6 in the last procedure, with an average duration of 12 months (range 2–24 months), and dilatation was performed as necessary before insertion of the prosthesis. The investigators obtained good results, with a success rate of 89% at 4 years of follow-up; 9% had minor early complications, 18% required an early replacement of the prosthesis, and no patients developed clinically significant recurrent stenosis.

In 2001 the authors published a series of 94 patients. The most frequent injury was Strasberg E1 to E3; all patients underwent sphincterotomy, and in 6 cases balloon dilatation was required before installation of the prosthesis. The number of prostheses ranged from 1 to 5 (5F–10F) and were left in situ for 8 months. At the end of treatment patients were assessed every 6 months for 3 years. There was a 2% complete failure of the prosthesis that required surgery, but no deaths or procedure-related complications were observed. The success rate at 2 years was 84%, which decreased to 76% at 3 years.[41]

As mentioned for the treatment of biliary fistulas, fully covered self-expandable prostheses are being evaluated for the treatment of benign strictures of the bile duct, with the advantage of providing better permeability, preventing occlusion, and thus reducing the number of procedures performed (**Fig. 5**). There are some prospective studies with small patient series that reflect good results with a mean follow-up of 1 year, with few complications.[24,26] More recent research has evaluated the use of bioabsorbable stents under development.[42]

The authors' center is participating in an international multicenter study that has just completed its recruitment phase of patients with benign strictures. This study will certainly provide important information regarding this topic.[43]

Recommendation

Even though the optimal number of prostheses placed, their size, the frequency of replacement, and the total optimal time in situ are not yet established, the data show that endoscopic therapy is successful in approximately 75% to 90% of cases

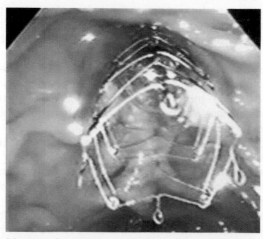

Fig. 5. Self-expandable stent for treatment of biliary common duct stenosis.

with a restenosis rate that does not exceed 20%, using a technique with a low percentage of morbidity and mortality.

SPECIAL CONSIDERATIONS FOR LIVER TRANSPLANTATION

Biliary complications after orthotopic liver transplantation (OLT) are present in up 20% of patients, of which the most common are stricture, bile leaks, stones, and dysfunction of the sphincter of Oddi. In this article only strictures and bile leaks are discussed.

The clinical presentation of post–liver transplant bile duct complications is often subtle, and the only clue for the diagnosis is commonly an asymptomatic increase in the baseline serum transaminase or bilirubin levels.

The use of endoscopy for biliary complications after OLT is influenced by the type of biliary reconstruction, the use of T-tubes, and the availability of subcutaneously placed limbs.[44–46]

Bile Leaks and Fistulas Associated with Liver Transplantation

Endoscopic management of bile leaks after transplantation follows the same principles described for the treatment of bile leaks secondary to laparoscopic cholecystectomy or biliary surgery. The bile leaks are associated with different aspects such as anastomosis, cystic duct, the T-tube tract and accessory conducts.[45] As a general

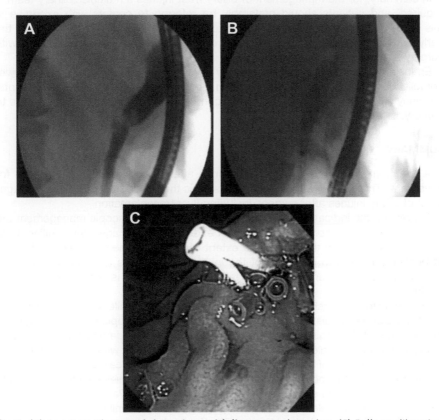

Fig. 6. (*A*) Anastomotic stenosis in patient with liver transplantation. (*B*) Balloon dilatation of biliary stenosis. (*C*) Multiple plastic stents installed in the biliary duct.

rule, drainage of related collection, endoscopic sphincterotomy, and stenting must be used for all cases.

If a T-tube cholangiogram identifies a minor leak, it can be conservatively managed, leaving the tube in place. Only refractory cases need endoscopic treatment.

Stricture Related to Liver Transplantation

Strictures are the most common complication associated with OLT, and are divided into early (within 60 days of transplantation), early to late (between 60 days and 1 year of transplantation), and late. Early strictures are mainly associated with technical errors in the anastomosis, whereas early to late and late strictures are often the consequence of vascular insufficiency.[44,45] The patients with early and early to late strictures respond well to temporary stent placement (3–6 months) and previous dilatation with balloon (**Fig. 6**). The latter case requires long-term follow-up, as the stricture can recur years after the transplantation. Late strictures respond well to the same therapy but the relapse rates can reach 40%, leading to a more complex treatment that includes repetitive balloon dilatation and a long-term (12–24 months) therapy with multiple (up to 8) large-diameter stents.[46,47] In recent years, self-expandable stents have been evaluated in these patients, with promising results. Randomized controlled trials are needed to confirm the greater effectiveness of metallic stents over plastic ones.[48–50]

In summary, for the management of biliary tract injuries a multidisciplinary team is required, and patients should preferably be referred to centers with expertise in this area. Endoscopic treatment is an excellent alternative to surgery in both the early and late postoperative stage, with results that are at least comparable with surgery.

Endoscopy, unlike surgery, is minimally invasive, reversible, and involves fewer complications, and should be considered in the treatment algorithm of these patients, for many as the only necessary therapeutic intervention and for some as a bridge to surgery.

SUMMARY

The treatment of common biliary duct injuries after surgery remains a challenge for physicians. This article reviews some endoscopic therapeutic options in the management of biliary injuries after surgery, including liver transplantation.

At present, the indications and contraindications for endoscopic management are based primarily on recommendations from experts. The management of biliary tract injuries will depend on the nature and extent of the injury, the presence or absence of biloma, and time to diagnosis of the injury. Most lesions are recognized in the postoperative period, and it is important that management is performed in referral centers.

According to the Strasberg classification, the lesions of the bile ducts may be divided into fistulas and stenosis. In biliary fistulas, the goal of endoscopic therapy is to reduce the pressure of the sphincter of Oddi. The alternatives include nasobiliary drainage, biliary sphincterotomy alone, placement of a prosthesis with or without sphincterotomy depending of the size of the fistula, and removal of a residual calculus if seen.

The objective in the management of biliary strictures is to relieve obstruction, and to prevent restenosis and secondary hepatocellular damage. Patients with a segment disconnection or complete transection injury should, by definition, undergo surgical management. Strasberg lesions E1 and E2 offer the best prognosis, and endoscopic management is possible. Most studies report good results with at least double insertion of a 10F prosthesis for a year and refills every 3 to 4 months. Self-expandable stents are being evaluated for this purpose.

The treatment of biliary injuries after surgery needs a multidisciplinary team. Endoscopic management is an available tool that has provided good results.

REFERENCES

1. Strasberg SM, Hertl M, Soper NJ. An analysis of the problem of biliary injury during laparoscopic cholecystectomy. J Am Coll Surg 1995;180(1):101–25.
2. McPartland KJ, Pomposelli J. Iatrogenic biliary injuries: classification, identification, and management. Surg Clin North Am 2008;88:1329–43.
3. Parlak E, Cicek B, Disibeyaz S, et al. Treatment of biliary leakages after cholecystectomy and importance of stricture development in the main bile duct injury. Turk J Gastroenterol 2005;16(1):21–8.
4. Kaffes AJ, Hourigan L, De LN. Impact of endoscopic intervention in 100 patients with suspected postcholecystectomy bile leak. Gastrointest Endosc 2005;61(2): 269–75.
5. Baron TH, Feitoza AB, Nagorney DM. Successful endoscopic treatment of a complete transection of the bile duct complicating laparoscopic cholecystectomy. Gastrointest Endosc 2003;57(6):765–9.
6. Sandha G, Bourke M, Haber G, et al. Endoscopic therapy for bile leak based on a new classification: results in 207 patients. Gastrointest Endosc 2004;60:567–74.
7. Isla AM, Griniatsos J, Karvounis E, et al. Advantages of laparoscopic stented choledochorrhaphy over T-tube placement. Br J Surg 2004;91(7):862–6.
8. Elboim CM, Goldman L, Hann L, et al. Significance of post-cholecystectomy subhepatic fluid collections. Ann Surg 1983;198:137.
9. Nuzzo G, Giulinate F, Giovannini I, et al. Advantages of multidisciplinary management of bile duct injuries occurring during cholecystectomy. Am J Surg 2008;195: 763–9.
10. Barkum AN, Rezieg M, Mehta SN, et al. Postcholecystectomy biliary leaks in the laparoscopic era: risk factors, presentation and management. Gastrointest Endosc 1997;45:277.
11. Bergman JJ, van den Brink GR, Rauws EA, et al. Treatment of bile duct lesions after laparoscopic cholecystectomy. Gut 1996;38:141.
12. Martin IJ, Bailey IS, Rhodes M, et al. Towards T-tube free laparoscopic bile duct exploration: a methodologic evolution during 300 consecutive procedures. Ann Surg 1998;228(1):29–34.
13. Bourke MJ, Elfont AB, Alhalel R, et al. Endoscopic management of postoperative bile leak in 85 patients. Gastrointest Endosc 1995;41:390.
14. Seitz U, Bapaye A, Bohnacker S, et al. Advances in therapeutic endoscopic treatment of common bile duct stones. World J Surg 1998;22(11):1133–44.
15. Navarrete C, Castillo C, Castillo P. Choledocholithiasis: percutaneous treatment. World J Surg 1998;22:1151–4.
16. Elmi F, Silverman WB. Nasobiliary tube management of postcholecystectomy bile leaks. J Clin Gastroenterol 2005;39(5):441–4.
17. Singh V, Singh G, Verma GR, et al. Endoscopic management of postcholecystectomy biliary leakage. Hepatobiliary Pancreat Dis Int 2010;9 409
18. Davids PH, Rauws EA, Tytgat GN, et al. Postoperative bile leakage: endoscopic management. Gut 1992;33:1118–22.
19. Foutch PG, Harlan JR, Hoefer M. Endoscopic therapy for patients with a postoperative biliary leaks. Gastrointest Endosc 1993;39:416–21.

20. Kozarek R, Gannan R, Baerg R, et al. Bile leak after laparoscopic cholecystectomy: diagnostic and therapeutic application of endoscopic retrograde cholangiopancreatography. Arch Intern Med 1992;152:1040–3.
21. De Palma GD, Gallaro G, Iuliano G, et al. Leaks from laparoscopic cholecystectomy. Hepatogastroenterology 2002;49:924–5.
22. Li S, Liang L, Peng B, et al. Bile leakage after hepatectomy for hepatolithiasis: risk factors and management. Surgery 2007;141:340–5.
23. Ryan ME, Geenen JE, Lehman GA, et al. Endoscopic intervention for biliary leaks after laparoscopic cholecystectomy: a multicenter review. Gastrointest Endosc 1998;47:261.
24. Navarrete C, Valdivieso E, Gobelet J. Biliary surgery complications including transplantation. In: Baron T, Kosarek R, Carr-Locke D, editors. ERCP. Philadelphia: Saunders Elsevier; 2008. p. 335–45.
25. Lubezky N, Konikoff FM, Rosin D, et al. Endoscopic sphincterotomy and temporary internal stenting for bile leaks following complex hepatic trauma. Br J Surg 2006;93:78–81.
26. van Berkel AM, Cahen DL, van Westerloo DJ, et al. Self-expanding metal stents in benign biliary strictures due to chronic pancreatitis. Endoscopy 2004;36(5):381–4.
27. Ahrendt S, Pitt HA. Surgical therapy of iatrogenic lesions of biliary tract. World J Surg 2001;25:1360–5.
28. De Palma G, Persico G, Sottile R, et al. Surgery or endoscopy for treatment of postcholecystectomy bile duct strictures? Am J Surg 2003;185:532–5.
29. Judah J, Draganov P. Endoscopic therapy of benign biliary strictures. World J Gastroenterol 2007;13:3531–9.
30. Davids PH, Tanks AK, Rauws EA, et al. Benign biliary strictures. Surgery or endoscopy? Ann Surg 1993;217:237.
31. Alves A, Farges O, Nicolet J, et al. Incidence and consequence of an hepatic artery injury in patients with postcholecystectomy bile duct strictures. Ann Surg 2003;238:93–6.
32. Wu Y, Linehan D. Bile duct injuries in the era of laparoscopic cholecystectomies. Surg Clin North Am 2010;90:787–802.
33. Lillemoe KD, Talamini MA, Wang BH, et al. Major bile duct injuries during laparoscopic cholecystectomy: follow-up after combined radiological and surgical management. Ann Surg 1997;225:459.
34. Walsh RM, Hennderson FM, Vogt DP, et al. Trends in bile duct injuries from laparoscopic cholecystectomy. J Gastrointest Surg 1998;2:458.
35. Nealon WH, Urrutia F. Long-term follow-up after bilioenteric anastomosis for benign bile duct stricture. Ann Surg 1996;223:639.
36. Lillemoe KD, Melton GB, Cameron JL, et al. Postoperative bile duct strictures: management and outcome in the 1990s. Ann Surg 2000;232:430–8.
37. Geenen DJ, Geenen JE, Hogen WJ, et al. Endoscopic therapy for benign bile duct strictures. Gastrointest Endosc 1992;38:12.
38. Bergman JJ, Burgemeister L, Bruno MJ, et al. Long-term follow-up after biliary stent placement for postoperative bile duct stenosis. Gastrointest Endosc 2001;54:154–61.
39. Costamagna G, Pandolfi M, Multignani M, et al. Long-term results of endoscopic management of postoperative bile duct strictures with increasing numbers of stents. Gastrointest Endosc 2001;54:162–8.
40. Fogel EL, Sherman S, Park SH, et al. Therapeutic biliary endoscopy. Endoscopy 2003;35(2):156–63.
41. Csendes A, Navarrete C, Burdiles P, et al. Treatment of common bile duct injuries during laparoscopic cholecystectomy: endoscopic and surgical management. World J Surg 2001;25:1346–51.

42. Ginsberg G, Cope C, Shah J, et al. In vivo evaluation of a new bioabsorbable self-expanding biliary stent. Gastrointest Endosc 2003;58(5):777–84.
43. Deviere J, Navarrete C, Costamagna G, et al. Preliminary results from a 187 patient multicenter prospective trial using metal stents for treatment of benign biliary strictures. In Programs and abstract of the Digestive Disease Week 2012. (Abstract #1298455).
44. Thuluvath PJ, Pfau PR, Kimmey MB, et al. Biliary complications after liver transplantation: the role of endoscopy. Endoscopy 2005;37(9):857–63.
45. Qian YB, Liu CL, Lo CM, et al. Risk factors for biliary complications after liver transplantation. Arch Surg 2004;139(10):1101–5.
46. Thuluvath PJ, Atassi T, Lee J. An endoscopic approach to biliary complications following orthotopic liver transplantation. Liver Int 2003;23(3):156–62.
47. Sibulesky L, Nguyen JH. Update on biliary strictures in liver transplants. Transplant Proc 2011;43:1760–4.
48. Traina M, Tarantino I, Barresi L, et al. Efficacy and safety of fully covered self-expandable metallic stents in biliary complications after liver transplantation: a preliminary study. Liver Transpl 2009;15:1493–8.
49. García-Pajares F, Sánchez-Antolín G, Pelayo SL, et al. Covered metal stents for the treatment of biliary complications after orthotopic liver transplantation. Transplant Proc 2010;42:2966.
50. Haapamäki C, Udd M, Halttunen J, et al. Endoscopic treatment of anastomotic biliary complications after liver transplantation using removable, covered, self-expandable metallic stents. Scand J Gastroenterol 2012;47:116–21.
51. Prat F, Pelletier G, Ponchon T, et al. What role can endoscopy play in the management of biliary complications after laparoscopic cholecystectomy? Endoscopy 1997;29:341–8.

Metal Stents for Hilar Lesions

Indu Srinivasan, MD[a], Michel Kahaleh, MD, AGAF[b,*]

KEYWORDS

- Hilar lesion • Metal stents • Self-expanding metal stent • Bismuth lesion
- Klatskin tumor

KEY POINTS

- Growing endoscopic inventions allow us to manage a variety of hilar lesions non-invasively by precluding surgery.
- Although metal stents have been offered for decades for unresectable hilar tumors, innovations such as cross-wired biliary SEMS, PDT, RFA, and EUS-guided biliary drainage have only recently been added to our arsenal.
- Moving forward, multicenter randomized control trials are required to prove their efficacy, thus establishing new standard of care.

INTRODUCTION

The hilar region is a complex one, containing the biliary, arterial, and venous structures. Stricture at this region can be caused by various benign and malignant causes. Some of the benign causes of hilar stricture include postsurgical injuries from cholecystectomy, liver transplantation or resection, and primary sclerosing cholangitis. Malignant hilar strictures are a group of heterogeneous tumors that include cholangiocarcinoma, tumors involving the hepatic confluence by direct extension from gallbladder, liver, and metastatic cancers. Cholangiocarcinoma is the most frequent cause of malignant hilar lesion, which accounts for only 3% of all the gastrointestinal malignancies. Perihilar cholangiocarcinoma, which involves the confluence of the right and left hepatic ducts, accounts for 60% to 70% of all the cholangiocarcinomas.[1]

Hilar tumor have been classified by Bismuth and colleagues[2] according to the type of involvement of the hepatic ducts. A type I lesion is located below the confluence of hepatic ducts, a type II lesion includes the confluence, type IIIa reaches the first radicals in the right and IIIb involves the radicals on the left, and type IV lesions are multicentric or involve the radicals on both sides. This classification is helpful not only in determining and planning surgical resection but also in endoscopic stent placement. Since originally described in 1965, various advances have been made in both interventional radiology and therapeutic endoscopy that have phenomenally changed the

[a] Department of Internal Medicine, Saint Vincent Hospital, Worcester, MA, USA; [b] Division of Gastroenterology and Hepatology, Department of Medicine, Weill Cornell Medical College, 1305 York Avenue, 4th Floor, New York, NY 10021, USA
* Corresponding author.
E-mail address: mkahaleh@gmail.com

Gastrointest Endoscopy Clin N Am 22 (2012) 555–565
doi:10.1016/j.giec.2012.05.009
1052-5157/12/$ – see front matter © 2012 Elsevier Inc. All rights reserved.

management of these tumors. This review focuses more on the growing indications of using metal stents in unresectable hilar tumors.

Hilar cancers, including cholangiocarcinoma, have an extremely poor prognosis with a 5-year survival rate of less than 10%.[1,3] The best prognosis with the best long-term survival has been in patients who undergo complete surgical resection with tumor-free margins.[1] This can unfortunately be performed in only 20%[2,4] of the patients. To increase the number of eligible candidates for surgical resection, a novel technique[5] with preoperative portal vein embolization to cause atrophy of the affected lobe and hypertrophy of normal tissue was evaluated in a bid to attain negative tumor margins. Once the decision for surgical resection is undertaken, the need for preoperative biliary drainage is still controversial, although some literature exists suggesting the need for preoperative biliary drainage via either ERCP or percutaneous transhepatic cholangiography (PTC) to decrease the perioperative mortality and morbidity from cholestasis. The rising complications from the instrumentation of the biliary tree, such as contamination, possible preoperative infection, and inflammation, further increasing the complexity of the surgery are the deal breakers. Further, there is an increasing incidence of tumor seeding associated with a percutaneous approach,[6] secondary to tumor manipulation with passage of a guide wire and a large catheter through the obstructing lesion resulting in the cellular disruption and seeding of the tumor cells through the biliary system. A meta-analysis[7] of 11 studies evaluating the benefit of preoperative biliary drainage with Hilar cholangiocarcinoma also concluded against routine performance of preoperative biliary drainage.

For patients with nonresectable tumors, as mentioned previously palliative biliary drainage is the treatment of choice. This can be performed either via surgery, endoscopic retrograde cholangiopancreatography (ERCP), or PTC. In general, surgical biliary-enteric bypass is not preferred[8,9] because of increased morbidity. With the rising complications of preoperative biliary drainage and surgical resection, the focus of treatment seems to have shifted to targeted and optimal endoscopic decompression for prolonged symptom-free survival.[3]

The consensus on this still remains controversial, as clinical trials have reported questionable benefits.[10]

BILIARY STENTS

Biliary stents were first introduced in 1979,[11] primarily for palliation of malignant biliary strictures, and then with the introduction of large-channel therapeutic duodenoscopes in 1982, endoscopic insertion of large-diameter plastic biliary endoprostheses became a reality. Higher risks of complications, such as occlusion and migration, associated with the plastic endoprosthesis led to the introduction of expandable metallic stents. Various studies conducted to compare the efficacy of plastic and metallic stents have demonstrated the supremacy of metallic stents[12,13] in treating malignant biliary strictures. Similarly, even for malignant hilar strictures self-expandable metal stents (SEMS) are preferred, owing to a decrease in frequency of endoscopic sessions and length of hospitalization, along with increased patency rates.[14,15] Despite their higher costs, they have been proven to be cost-effective in patients who survive more than 4 to 6 months. A retrospective study[3] conducted over 10 years also demonstrated the efficacy of SEMS in palliation of hilar cholangiocarcinoma. Fifty-two metal stent were inserted in 36 patients; 97% of the cases obtained successful internal biliary drainage. Median patency of the stents was 169 days with a low complication rate of 14%. The most interesting observation of the study was that 69% of patients did not require any further biliary reinterventions after initial metal stent placement. Plastic stents are still being used, especially when the diagnosis of cancer is not confirmed, or the patient is a surgical candidate, or is receiving photodynamic therapy[16,17] or brachytherapy.[18]

Experts have recommended using uncovered SEMS[3] for lesions in the intrahepatic and hilar regions to avoid blocking the drainage of other intrahepatic segments with covered SEMS, as it would lead to segmental cholangitis. Higher rates of migration[19,20] associated with covered SEMS may possibly be yet another reason for advocating uncovered stents.

TECHNIQUE

To perform ERCP in these patients with obstruction at the hilar level, it is necessary to do so only after reviewing the prerequisite cross-sectional images to help us delineate the anatomy before proceeding with the procedure (**Fig. 1**). On reaching the desired segment that needs to be drained based on our imaging, selective cannulation should be performed by advancing the guide wire into the segment over which the catheter is advanced and the contrast is injected proximal to the obstruction (**Fig. 2**). Contrasts should be injected only in the segments that are planned to be drained and only healthy segments of the liver should be drained. After the initial cannulation, biliary sphincterotomy is performed and the stricture is dilated using either the balloon or dilating catheter and the stents are placed (**Fig. 3**). During this procedure, choledochoscopy can also be performed to assess and sample the stricture.

The debate of bilateral versus unilateral stenting of the hilar region is still contented, as various studies have revealed conflicting data. Bilateral drainage is a more physiologic than unilateral drainage, but is technically more demanding.[21,22] This concept of placing multiple stents for obtaining maximal drainage has been supported by many studies[23,24] that have proven improvement in clinical symptoms and survival. This was challenged by a few other studies.[25,26] A randomized trial[27] of 157 patients revealed endoscopic success of unilateral over bilateral stenting (89% vs 77%, $P = .041$) associated with lower rate of complication (27% vs 19%, $P = .026$) without a change in median survival. Although the verdict is still debatable, in cases of contralateral cholangitis or persistent jaundice with unilateral stenting, then bilateral stenting is mandated. Owing to the difficulties in obtaining the idealistic maximal biliary drainage, different methods have been described in the literature, such as selective placement of guide wires on both sides of the intrahepatic biliary tree[28]: parallel stent deployment, where after guide wire placement on both sides, a plastic stent is placed on first side and SEMS is deployed on the other side, the plastic stent is removed and then exchanged with SEMS; temporary placement of a plastic stent inside the metallic stent to prevent it from fully expanding[29];

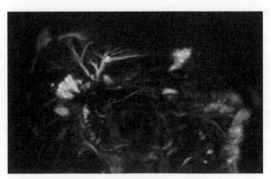

Fig. 1. MRI-MRCP of hilar lesion with proximal biliary dilation.

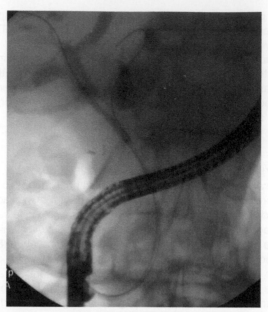

Fig. 2. Fluoroscopy of a Klastkin cancer with access in the right hepatic duct and left hepatic duct followed by selective dilation (Patient A).

deployment of a second SEMS through the first SEMS after disrupting the interstices[3]; and use of "open mesh" SEMS with 8-mm interstices in the central section realizing a T-shaped[30] or Y-shaped[31] configuration. With multiple stent placements, there is always a risk of potential entanglement of 2 guide wires, dislodgement of the stents, and difficulty of exact positioning of both the stents to ensure maximal drainage. In an attempt to overcome some of these difficulties, Lee and colleagues[31] conducted a pilot study to evaluate the efficacy of a newly designed Y stent. This was a self-expandable nitinol stent with a central part of Y stent developed as an open mesh to allow for a second stent (Z stent) to be introduced into the contralateral bile duct. Lee and colleagues[31] studied this technique in 10 patients, of whom 8 achieved technical success (**Fig. 4**). Although there were no immediate complications, stent occlusion developed in 25% of the cases. Recently, SEMS with an easily expandable mid-portion have been evaluated for hilar cholangiocarcinoma. The first SEMS placed has 2 spiral markings in 25 mm of the central portion and has 4 spot markings on both ends (BONASTENT M-Hilar; Standard Sci Tech Inc., Seoul, South Korea). The whole stent has a hook and cross-wired structure with the area between the central spiral markings containing only a cross-wired structured to facilitate expansion and deployment of the second stent. Park and colleagues[32] conducted a multicenter trial with these latest designed stents on 35 patients. They reported an overall success rate of bilateral placement as 33% with an 82% success rate in a single session. Their 6% complication rate compared favorably with the previously reported complication rate.

A retrospective multicenter trial was conducted by Paik and colleagues[33] to compare the endoscopic and percutaneous approaches in the palliative treatment of type III and type IV carcinomas by using biliary SEMS. A total of 85 patients were included in the study; 45 underwent endoscopic stent placement and 41 underwent the percutaneous approach. Effective relief of cholestasis was achieved in 92.7% of the percutaneous group, whereas in the endoscopic group it was only 77.3%. Further,

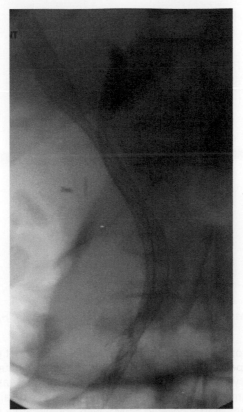

Fig. 3. Fluoroscopy of a Klastkin cancer with uncovered metal stents placed in the right hepatic duct and left hepatic ducts (Patient A).

the mean duration of hospital stay was significantly shorter in the endoscopic group. There was no significant difference in the duration of the patency of the stents or overall survival rates. Based on their findings, the investigators recommended that the percutaneous approach with biliary SEMS should be the initial approach of palliation in type III and type IV.

However, recent endoscopic innovations[34] have facilitated the ease with which specific bile ducts can be stented and have further decreased the risk of cholangitis. This, combined with the increased risk of hemorrhage, tumor seeding, and the psychological impact of an external drain on a patient, has reduced its role in the management to that of either a backup option or when a combined approach is required.

Usually after a failed ERCP procedure, percutaneous transhepatic biliary drainage (PTBD) is performed as a salvage step. Once the initial drainage is obtained, then either an external drain can be placed or a PTBD-ERCP rendezvous can be performed, which includes inserting of a guide wire across the percutaneous drainage catheter into the bile duct that is caught by a snare, which is subsequently pulled into the working channel of the duodenoscope and can be used to guide catheter insertion. This has paved the way for endoscopic ultrasound-guided biliary drainage (EUSBD).

With the introduction of linear echoendoscopes in 1990s, the era of therapeutic EUS had arrived. Since 2001,[35] when it was first published, various studies have been reported but unfortunately the published data on this remain sparse and most of the

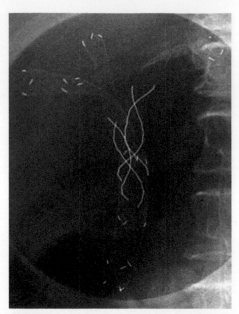

Fig. 4. Cross-wired metal stents at the hilum. (*Courtesy of* Dr Moon JH, MD, PhD, Bucheon, Korea.)

studies have been done on plastic stents. Of the few studies that were conducted on metal stents, a prospective feasibility study by Park and colleagues[36] on 14 patients with malignant biliary obstruction showed an initial success rate of 100% with 1 patient requiring reintervention. In 2011, Horaguchi and colleagues[37] from Japan described deployment of fully covered SEMS with antimigratory fins in 5 patients in a single session. One of the most interesting applications of EUSBD for hilar lesions is for patients with altered anatomy, such as s/p Whipple with recurrence at the confluence, the ability to provide selective and targeted biliary decompression of the left biliary tree (**Figs. 5–8**) provides a dramatic improvement in terms of quality of life in patients previously receiving percutaneous drains.

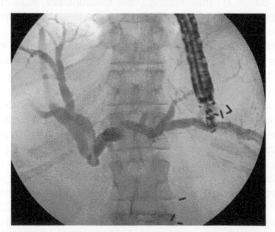

Fig. 5. EUS-guided injection of the left hepatic duct in a patient with recurrent pancreatic cancer s/p Whipple, showing dilated right and left hepatic duct above the confluence (Patient B).

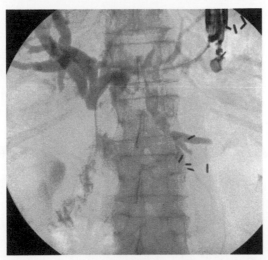

Fig. 6. EUS-guided advancement of the wire into the stricture located at the confluence and extending to the hepatico-jejunostomy (Patient B).

Although results look extremely promising, more data and experience are required in this field. For performing this technique, individuals need to be trained in both EUS and ERCP. This intervention is currently restricted to a few tertiary-level centers. Major complications associated with this technique include perforation, biliary leak with peritonitis, and bleeding, which are uncommon in expert hands.

More recently, photodynamic therapy (PDT) and radiofrequency ablation (RFA) have also emerged as adjuvant therapies, along with stent placement in unresectable cholangiocarcinoma to increase both stent patency and life expectancy. PDT is a 2-step process that involves injecting of an intravenous porphyrin photosensitizer followed by endoscopic application of nonthermal laser light of specific wavelength to the

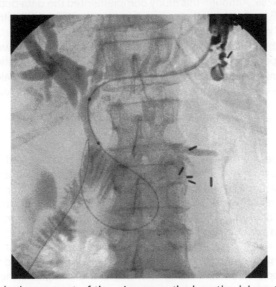

Fig. 7. EUS-guided advancement of the wire across the hepatico-jejunostomy (Patient B).

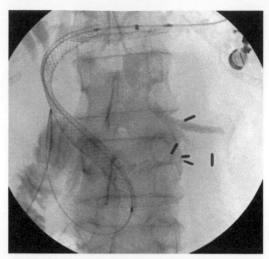

Fig. 8. EUS-guided placement of an uncovered metal stent draining the left hepatic duct (Patient B).

tumor bed, resulting in generation of oxygen free radicals. Various studies[16,38] have demonstrated the efficacy of this combined approach. A pilot study of 9 patients by Ortner and colleagues[16] revealed significantly longer survival (493 vs 93 days) along with improved biliary drainage and quality of life when compared with patients who solely underwent stenting. This was subsequently confirmed in numerous other trials. Subsequently, in 2008, Kahaleh and colleagues[39] compared stenting alone with the combined effect of stenting with PDT in 48 patients. Kaplan-Meier analysis demonstrated an improved survival benefit in the combination therapy as opposed to the stenting group. The mortality in the PDT group at the end of 3 months, 6 months, and 12 months was 0%, 16%, and 56%, whereas in the stent group mortality was 28%, 52%, and 82%. Although this study complemented the data published by Ortner and colleagues,[16] it was not entirely clear that the benefit was directly related to PDT or the number of endoscopic sessions.

RFA has also been described in the literature as one of the novel techniques of improving life expectancy. In a study conducted in China on 11 patients (stage III or IV) who underwent percutaneous transhepatic cholangiographic drainage initially followed by multiple electrodes RFA, a follow-up scan in 6 months revealed 35% reduction in tumor size with a mean survival rate of 18 months.

COMPLICATIONS

The past 2 decades have seen tremendous strides being made in the field of endoscopy, changing it from a diagnostic tool to a therapeutic one. Although most endoscopists are well trained and have a cannulation rate of greater than 85%, with experts reaching as high as 95%,[40] selective endoscopic stenting into the appropriate bile duct is still a challenge.[24] This is one of the limitations to performing an effective biliary drainage in hilar cholangiocarcinoma. Cholangitis from the procedure-related complications of metal stent insertion in these patients is low.[15] Studies conducted in the past suggested that minimizing the contrast into the obstructed biliary segments to avoid biliary opacification,[41] along with bilateral drainage, is the most probable reason for this low risk.

Stent occlusion is one of the common complications of the procedure and is probably the single most important factor in predicting the risk of biliary reintervention. The various etiologies for stent occlusion in uncovered SEMS include epithelial overgrowth resulting in inflammation and obstruction,[42,43] whereas in covered SEMS tumor ingrowth or overgrowth or overwhelming tissue burden can contribute to biliary sludge and occlusion.[44] The overall occlusion rates in studies have been reported in 18% to 24%[15] of the cases. Most cases of occlusion are managed by inserting a plastic stent through the metal stent.

Further, unlike plastic stents, uncovered metal stents cannot be extracted once they are deployed, as they become embedded[45] in the tumor bed. Thus, they should be used carefully and only after confirming the presence of unresectable malignancy.

SUMMARY

We are currently in an exciting phase of growing endoscopic inventions that allow us to manage a host of biliary conditions by precluding surgery or invasive procedures. Although use of metal stents in hilar lesions has been offered for decades, innovations such as cross-wired biliary SEMS, PDT, RFA, and EUSBD have added to our arsenal. Moving forward, multicenter randomized control trials are required to prove their efficacy and alter our standard of care.

ACKNOWLEDGMENTS

I would like to acknowledge my radiology technician, Steven Zerbo, for his assistance in providing the figures.

REFERENCES

1. Nakeeb A, Pitt HA, Sohn TA, et al. Cholangiocarcinoma. A spectrum of intrahepatic, perihilar, and distal tumors. Ann Surg 1996;224(4):463–73 [discussion: 473–5].
2. Bismuth H, Castaing D, Traynor O. Resection or palliation: priority of surgery in the treatment of hilar cancer. World J Surg 1988;12(1):39–47.
3. Cheng JL, Bruno MJ, Bergman JJ, et al. Endoscopic palliation of patients with biliary obstruction caused by nonresectable hilar cholangiocarcinoma: efficacy of self-expandable metallic wallstents. Gastrointest Endosc 2002;56(1):33–9.
4. Chamberlain RS, Blumgart LH. Hilar cholangiocarcinoma: a review and commentary. Ann Surg Oncol 2000;7(1):55–66.
5. Palavecino M, Abdalla EK, Madoff DC, et al. Portal vein embolization in hilar cholangiocarcinoma. Surg Oncol Clin N Am 2009;18(2):257–67, viii.
6. Chapman WC, Sharp KW, Weaver F, et al. Tumor seeding from percutaneous biliary catheters. Ann Surg 1989;209(6):708–13 [discussion: 713–5].
7. Liu F, Li Y, Wei Y, et al. Preoperative biliary drainage before resection for hilar cholangiocarcinoma: whether or not? A systematic review. Dig Dis Sci 2011; 56(3):663–72.
8. Andersen JR, Sørensen SM, Kruse A, et al. Randomised trial of endoscopic endoprosthesis versus operative bypass in malignant obstructive jaundice. Gut 1989;30(8):1132–5.
9. Smith AC, Dowsett JF, Russell RC, et al. Randomised trial of endoscopic stenting versus surgical bypass in malignant low bileduct obstruction. Lancet 1994; 344(8938):1655–60.
10. Kawakami H, Kondo S, Kuwatani M, et al. Preoperative biliary drainage for hilar cholangiocarcinoma: which stent should be selected? J Hepatobiliary Pancreat Sci 2011;18(5):630–5.

11. Soehendra N, Reynders-Frederix V. [Palliative biliary duct drainage. A new method for endoscopic introduction of a new drain]. Dtsch Med Wochenschr 1979;104(6):206–7 [in German].

12. Davids PH, Groen AK, Rauws EA, et al. Randomised trial of self-expanding metal stents versus polyethylene stents for distal malignant biliary obstruction. Lancet 1992;340(8834–8835):1488–92.

13. Soderlund C, Linder S. Covered metal versus plastic stents for malignant common bile duct stenosis: a prospective, randomized, controlled trial. Gastrointest Endosc 2006;63(7):986–95.

14. Zhou J, Tang ZY, Wu ZQ, et al. Factors influencing survival in hepatocellular carcinoma patients with macroscopic portal vein tumor thrombosis after surgery, with special reference to time dependency: a single-center experience of 381 cases. Hepatogastroenterology 2006;53(68):275–80.

15. Wagner HJ, Knyrim K, Vakil N, et al. Plastic endoprostheses versus metal stents in the palliative treatment of malignant hilar biliary obstruction. A prospective and randomized trial. Endoscopy 1993;25(3):213–8.

16. Ortner ME, Caca K, Berr F, et al. Successful photodynamic therapy for nonresectable cholangiocarcinoma: a randomized prospective study. Gastroenterology 2003;125(5):1355–63.

17. Harewood GC, Baron TH, Rumalla A, et al. Pilot study to assess patient outcomes following endoscopic application of photodynamic therapy for advanced cholangiocarcinoma. J Gastroenterol Hepatol 2005;20(3):415–20.

18. Simmons DT, Baron TH, Petersen BT, et al. A novel endoscopic approach to brachytherapy in the management of hilar cholangiocarcinoma. Am J Gastroenterol 2006;101(8):1792–6.

19. Wamsteker EJ, Elta GH. Migration of covered biliary self-expanding metallic stents in two patients with malignant biliary obstruction. Gastrointest Endosc 2003;58(5):792–3.

20. Matsushita M, Takakuwa H, Nishio A, et al. Open-biopsy-forceps technique for endoscopic removal of distally migrated and impacted biliary metallic stents. Gastrointest Endosc 2003;58(6):924–7.

21. Sherman S. Endoscopic drainage of malignant hilar obstruction: is one biliary stent enough or should we work to place two? Gastrointest Endosc 2001;53(6):681–4.

22. Polydorou AA, Chisholm EM, Romanos AA, et al. A comparison of right versus left hepatic duct endoprosthesis insertion in malignant hilar biliary obstruction. Endoscopy 1989;21(6):266–71.

23. Arvanitakis M, Van Laethem JL, Pouzere S, et al. Predictive factors for survival in patients with inoperable Klatskin tumors. Hepatogastroenterology 2006;53(67):21–7.

24. Deviere J, Baize M, de Toeuf J, et al. Long-term follow-up of patients with hilar malignant stricture treated by endoscopic internal biliary drainage. Gastrointest Endosc 1988;34(2):95–101.

25. De Palma GD, Pezzullo A, Rega M, et al. Unilateral placement of metallic stents for malignant hilar obstruction: a prospective study. Gastrointest Endosc 2003; 58(1):50–3.

26. Freeman ML, Overby C. Selective MRCP and CT-targeted drainage of malignant hilar biliary obstruction with self-expanding metallic stents. Gastrointest Endosc 2003;58(1):41–9.

27. De Palma GD, Galloro G, Siciliano S, et al. Unilateral versus bilateral endoscopic hepatic duct drainage in patients with malignant hilar biliary obstruction: results of a prospective, randomized, and controlled study. Gastrointest Endosc 2001; 53(6):547–53.

28. Dumas R, Demuth N, Buckley M, et al. Endoscopic bilateral metal stent placement for malignant hilar stenoses: identification of optimal technique. Gastrointest Endosc 2000;51(3):334–8.

29. Hookey LC, Le Moine O, Deviere J. Use of a temporary plastic stent to facilitate the placement of multiple self-expanding metal stents in malignant biliary hilar strictures. Gastrointest Endosc 2005;62(4):605–9.

30. Kim CW, Park AW, Won JW, et al. T-configured dual stent placement in malignant biliary hilar duct obstructions with a newly designed stent. J Vasc Interv Radiol 2004;15(7):713–7.

31. Lee JH, Kang DH, Kim JY, et al. Endoscopic bilateral metal stent placement for advanced hilar cholangiocarcinoma: a pilot study of a newly designed Y stent. Gastrointest Endosc 2007;66(2):364–9.

32. Park do H, Lee SS, Moon JH, et al. Newly designed stent for endoscopic bilateral stent-in-stent placement of metallic stents in patients with malignant hilar biliary strictures: multicenter prospective feasibility study (with videos). Gastrointest Endosc 2009;69(7):1357–60.

33. Paik WH, Park YS, Hwang JH, et al. Palliative treatment with self-expandable metallic stents in patients with advanced type III or IV hilar cholangiocarcinoma: a percutaneous versus endoscopic approach. Gastrointest Endosc 2009;69(1):55–62.

34. Knyrim K, Wagner HJ, Pausch J, et al. A prospective, randomized, controlled trial of metal stents for malignant obstruction of the common bile duct. Endoscopy 1993;25(3):207–12.

35. Giovannini M, Moutardier V, Pesenti C, et al. Endoscopic ultrasound-guided bilioduodenal anastomosis: a new technique for biliary drainage. Endoscopy 2001; 33(10):898–900.

36. Park do H, Koo JE, Oh J, et al. EUS-guided biliary drainage with one-step placement of a fully covered metal stent for malignant biliary obstruction: a prospective feasibility study. Am J Gastroenterol 2009;104(9):2168–74.

37. Horaguchi J, Fujita N, Noda Y, et al. One-step placement of a fully-covered metal stent in endosonography-guided biliary drainage for malignant biliary obstruction. Intern Med 2011;50(19):2089–93.

38. Zoepf T, Jakobs R, Arnold JC, et al. Palliation of nonresectable bile duct cancer: improved survival after photodynamic therapy. Am J Gastroenterol 2005;100(11): 2426–30.

39. Kahaleh M, Mishra R, Shami VM, et al. Unresectable cholangiocarcinoma: comparison of survival in biliary stenting alone versus stenting with photodynamic therapy. Clin Gastroenterol Hepatol 2008;6(3):290–7.

40. Baron TH, Petersen BT, Mergener K, et al. Quality indicators for endoscopic retrograde cholangiopancreatography. Gastrointest Endosc 2006;63(Suppl 4):S29–34.

41. Chang WH, Kortan P, Haber GB. Outcome in patients with bifurcation tumors who undergo unilateral versus bilateral hepatic duct drainage. Gastrointest Endosc 1998;47(5):354–62.

42. Smith MT, Sherman S, Lehman GA. Endoscopic management of benign strictures of the biliary tree. Endoscopy 1995;27(3):253–66.

43. Irving JD, Adam A, Dick R, et al. Gianturco expandable metallic biliary stents: results of a European clinical trial. Radiology 1989;172(2):321–6.

44. Bezzi M, Zolovkins A, Cantisani V, et al. New ePTFE/FEP-covered stent in the palliative treatment of malignant biliary obstruction. J Vasc Interv Radiol 2002; 13(6):581–9.

45. Familiari P, Bulajic M, Mutignani M, et al. Endoscopic removal of malfunctioning biliary self-expandable metallic stents. Gastrointest Endosc 2005;62(6):903–10.

Complications of Endoscopic Retrograde Cholangiopancreatography

Avoidance and Management

Martin L. Freeman, MD

KEYWORDS

- Endoscopic retrograde cholangiopancreatography • ERCP
- Post-ERCP pancreatitis • Hemorrhage • Perforation • Complications

KEY POINTS

- Complications occur after 5% to 10% of endoscopic retrograde cholangiopancreatography (ERCP).
- Risk factors for post-ERCP pancreatitis include patient-related as well as procedure-related variables.
- Placement of prophylactic pancreatic stents is effective, reducing risk of pancreatitis after ERCP.
- Hemorrhage after sphincterotomy is primarily related to coagulation defects, but can be treated by endoscopic hemostasis techniques.
- Perforation can involve bowel wall, sphincterotomy, or guidewire; early recognition and management are key to satisfactory outcomes.
- Endoscopist experience is reflected in complication rates.

OVERVIEW

Endoscopic retrograde cholangiopancreatography (ERCP) is now almost exclusively a therapeutic modality for pancreatic as well as biliary disorders. ERCP alone or with associated pancreatic and biliary therapy can cause a spectrum of complications, including pancreatitis, hemorrhage, perforation, and cardiopulmonary events (**Box 1**). These complications can range from mild (defined as requiring 3 or fewer nights' hospitalization), to severe (resulting in extended hospitalization, requiring surgical intervention, and resulting in permanent disability or even death). Understanding of complications of ERCP has progressed substantially in the past decade, including widespread adoption of standardized consensus-based definitions of complications,[1] large multi-center multivariate studies that have permitted clearer understanding of patient and

Division of Gastroenterology, Hepatology and Nutrition, University of Minnesota, MMC 36, 406 Harvard Street SE, Minneapolis, MN 55455, USA
E-mail address: freem020@umn.edu

Gastrointest Endoscopy Clin N Am 22 (2012) 567–586
doi:10.1016/j.giec.2012.05.001
1052-5157/12/$ – see front matter © 2012 Elsevier Inc. All rights reserved.

> **Box 1**
> **Complications of ERCP**
>
> - Pancreatitis
> - Hemorrhage
> - Perforation
> - Cholangitis
> - Cholecystitis
> - Stent-related
> - Cardiopulmonary
> - Miscellaneous

technique-related risk factors for complications,[2–9] and introduction of new technical approaches to minimize risks of ERCP.

CONSENSUS-BASED DEFINITIONS OF COMPLICATIONS AND OTHER NEGATIVE OUTCOMES

Standardized definitions for complications of sphincterotomy were introduced in 1991[1] and are still widely used for therapeutic ERCP in general (**Table 1**). Severity is assessed primarily by length of hospital stay, and intervention required to treat the complications. Universal consensus-based definitions have allowed valid comparisons of outcomes of therapeutic ERCP in various settings. There is an increasing awareness of the entire spectrum of outcomes, including technical failures, ineffectiveness of the procedure in resolving the presenting clinical problem, long-term sequelae, costs, extended hospitalization, and patient (dis)satisfaction. The term complications has to some degree been supplanted by the terms adverse events and unplanned events. A successful procedure with a minor or even a moderate complication may sometimes be a preferable outcome to a failed procedure attempt without any obvious complication: the kinds of advanced procedures discussed elsewhere in this issue show the complexity of therapeutics now performed at ERCP, often substituting for major surgery or interventional radiologic procedures, all with their own risk of morbidity and mortality, as well as resource use.

VARIATIONS IN COMPLICATION RATES BETWEEN STUDIES

Complication rates of ERCP vary widely, even between apparently similar prospective studies. Variation is substantial. For example, in 1 large prospective study, post-ERCP pancreatitis rates were reported at 0.74% for diagnostic ERCP, and 1.4% for therapeutic ERCP, respectively[7]; in another similar study, postprocedure pancreatitis rates were 5.1% (7-fold higher) for diagnostic ERCP and 6.9% (5-fold higher) for therapeutic ERCP.[3] Possible reasons for such wide variation in reported complication rates include variation in (1) definitions; (2) thoroughness of protocol for detection of complications; (3) patient population with attendant risk factors; and (4) differences in spectrum of technical approach such as use of pancreatic stents, or different end points of therapy.

Multivariable analysis is a useful statistical method to identify and quantify the effect of multiple potentially confounding risk factors. However, such analysis is not absolute because potentially key risk factors may or may not have been analyzed. In addition, sample size must be large for valid multivariable analysis, to avoid overfitting of the

Table 1
Consensus definitions for the major complications of ERCP

	Mild	Moderate	Severe
Pancreatitis	Clinical pancreatitis, amylase at least 3 times normal at more that 24 h after the procedure, requiring admission or prolongation of planned admission to 2–3 d	Pancreatitis requiring hospitalization of 4–10 d	Hospitalization for more than 10 d, pseudocyst, or intervention (percutaneous drainage or surgery)
Bleeding	Clinical (ie, not just endoscopic) evidence of bleeding, hemoglobin drop <3 g, no transfusion	Transfusion (4 units or less), no angiographic intervention or surgery	Transfusion 5 units or more, or intervention (angiographic or surgical)
Perforation	Possible, or only slight leak of fluid or contrast, treatable by fluids and suction for ≤3 d	Any definite perforation treated medically 4–10 d	Medical treatment of more than 10 d, or intervention (percutaneous or surgical)
Infection (cholangitis)	>38°C for 24–48 h	Febrile or septic illness requiring more than 3 d of hospital treatment or percutaneous intervention	Septic shock or surgery

Any intensive care unit admission after a procedure grades the complication as severe.
Other rarer complications can be graded by length of needed hospitalization.
From Cotton PB, Lehman G, Vennes JA, et al. Endoscopic sphincterotomy complications and their management: an attempt at consensus. Gastrointest Endosc 1991;37:383–91; with permission.

model and thus suggesting spurious associations. Only a few multicenter studies have included more than 1000 patients. **Tables 2–4** present summaries of risk factors for complications of therapeutic and diagnostic ERCP based on published multivariate analyses.

COMPLICATIONS OF DIAGNOSTIC AND THERAPEUTIC ERCP

Prospective series of ERCP generally report an overall short-term complication rate of approximately 5% to 10%.[2–9] Certain patterns emerge from most studies. There is a particularly high rate of complications (up to 20% or more, primarily pancreatitis, with up to 5% severe complications) for ERCP and sphincterotomy for suspected sphincter of Oddi dysfunction. In contrast, there is a consistently low complication rate for routine bile duct stone extraction (<5% in most series).[2] Hemorrhage occurs primarily after sphincterotomy, and primarily in patients with bile duct stones, coagulopathy, and acute cholangitis. Cholangitis occurs mostly after ERCP in patients with malignant biliary obstruction or failed drainage, or after stent malfunction or occlusion. Perforation occurs primarily after sphincterotomy, or is endoscope-related, but risk factors are more difficult to determine.

Risk factors for overall complications of ERCP and sphincterotomy by multivariable analyses are shown in **Table 2**. Although relevant studies are heterogeneous and sometimes omit potentially key risk factors, several patterns are apparent. Indication of suspected sphincter of Oddi dysfunction is a significant risk factor; technical factors, likely related to specific expertise or approach of the endoscopist and center, are also significant risk factors for overall complications. These technical factors include difficult cannulation, use of precut or access papillotomy to gain bile duct entry, failure to achieve biliary drainage, and use of simultaneous or subsequent percutaneous biliary drainage for otherwise failed endoscopic cannulation. In turn, the ERCP case volume of the endoscopists or medical centers, when examined, has almost always been a significant factor in complications by both univariate or multivariable analysis.[2–9] Death from ERCP is rare (<0.5%), but is most often caused by cardiopulmonary complications. It is unclear whether the increasing use of anesthesia services for monitored anesthesia care or general anesthesia during ERCP has affected the cardiopulmonary complication rate.

Contrary to intuition and commonly held beliefs, risk factors found not to be significant for overall complications include older age or increased number of coexisting

Table 2		
Risk factors for overall complications of ERCP in multivariate analyses		
Definite[a]	**Maybe[b]**	**No[c]**
Suspected sphincter of Oddi dysfunction	Young age	Comorbid illness
Cirrhosis	Pancreatic contrast injection	Small common bile duct diameter
Difficult cannulation	Failed biliary drainage	Female sex
Precut sphincterotomy	Trainee involvement	Billroth II
Percutaneous biliary access		Periampullary diverticulum
Lower ERCP case volume		

[a] Significant by multivariate analysis in most studies.
[b] Significant by univariate analysis only in most studies.
[c] Not significant by multivariate analysis in any study.

Table 3
Risk factors for post-ERCP pancreatitis in multivariate analyses

Definite[a]	Maybe[b]	No[c]
Suspected sphincter of Oddi dysfunction	Female sex	Small common bile duct diameter
Young age	Acinarization	Sphincter of Oddi manometry
Normal bilirubin	Absence of common bile duct stone	Biliary sphincterotomy
History of post-ERCP pancreatitis	Lower ERCP case volume	
Difficult or failed cannulation	Trainee involvement	
Pancreatic duct injection		
Pancreatic guidewire placement		
Pancreatic tissue sampling by any means		
Pancreatic sphincterotomy (especially minor papilla)		
Balloon dilation of intact biliary sphincter		
Precut sphincterotomy		

[a] Significant by multivariate analysis in most studies.
[b] Significant by univariate analysis only in most studies.
[c] Not significant by multivariate analysis in any study.

medical conditions; on the contrary, younger age generally increases the risk both by univariate and multivariate analysis, smaller bile duct diameter, and anatomic variants such as periampullary diverticulum or Billroth II gastrectomy, although they do increase technical difficulty for the endoscopist.[2–9]

POST-ERCP PANCREATITIS

Pancreatitis is the most common complication of ERCP, with reported rates varying from 1% to 40%, with a rate of about 5% being most typical.[2–9] In the Cotton consensus classification,[1] post-ERCP pancreatitis is defined as clinical syndrome consistent with pancreatitis (ie, new or worsened abdominal pain) with an amylase level at least 3 times normal at more than 24 hours after the procedure, and requiring

Table 4
Risk factors for hemorrhage after endoscopic sphincterotomy in multivariate analyses

Definite[a]	Maybe[b]	No[c]
Coagulopathy	Cirrhosis	Aspirin or nonsteroidal antiinflammatory drug
Anticoagulation <3 d after ERCP	Dilated common bile duct	Ampullary tumor
Cholangitis before ERCP	Common bile duct stone	Longer sphincterotomy
Bleeding during sphincterotomy	Periampullary diverticulum	Extension of previous sphincterotomy
Lower ERCP case volume	Precut sphincterotomy	

[a] Significant by multivariate analysis in most studies.
[b] Significant by univariate analysis only in most studies.
[c] Not significant by multivariate analysis in any study.

more than 1 night of hospitalization (see **Table 1**). More difficult to classify according to consensus definitions are patients with postprocedural abdominal pain and increase of serum lipase level to more than 3 times normal simultaneous with amylase level increase to less than 3 times upper limit of normal, or those with dramatic lipase increases but minimal symptoms that are not clearly suggestive of clinical pancreatitis. This situation is particularly true of patients with chronic pain in whom postprocedural pain can be difficult to assess and may persist despite normal pancreatic enzymes, or may persist long after pancreatic enzymes have normalized, and without imaging evidence of acute pancreatitis.

Risk Factors for Post-ERCP Pancreatitis Related to the Patient

Mechanical, chemical, hydrostatic, enzymatic, microbiologic, and thermal injury have all been postulated as potential mechanisms of injury to the pancreas during ERCP and endoscopic sphincterotomy. Although the relative contribution of these factors is not known, recent multivariate analyses have helped to identify the clinical patient-related and procedure-related factors that are independently associated with pancreatitis. The risk of post-ERCP pancreatitis is determined at least as much by the characteristics of the patient as by endoscopic techniques or maneuvers (see **Table 3**). Factors found to be significant in 1 or more major studies include younger age, indication of suspected sphincter of Oddi dysfunction, history of previous post-ERCP pancreatitis, and normal serum bilirubin level.[2–9] Women may be at increased risk, but it is difficult to determine the confounding effect of sphincter of Oddi dysfunction, a condition that occurs almost exclusively in women. In 1 meta-analysis, female gender was clearly a risk,[10] and women account for most cases of severe or fatal post-ERCP pancreatitis.[2,11,12]

Sphincter of Oddi dysfunction, a controversial syndrome that is primarily suspected in women with postcholecystectomy abdominal pain, poses a formidable risk for pancreatitis after any kind of ERCP, whether diagnostic, manometric, or therapeutic. The risk of post-ERCP pancreatitis triples to 10% to 30% in patients with suspected sphincter of Oddi dysfunction.[2–5] The reason for heightened susceptibility in these patients remains unknown. Contrary to widely held opinion, sphincter of Oddi manometry is not the culprit. Multivariable analyses all show that empiric biliary sphincterotomy or even diagnostic ERCP has similarly high risk.[3] With the widespread use of aspiration instead of conventional perfusion manometry catheters, the risk of manometry has probably been reduced to that of cannulation with any other ERCP accessory. Most previous studies linking manometry with risk have been from tertiary centers in which manometry is always performed in patients with suspected sphincter of Oddi dysfunction, thus suggesting guilt by association rather than cause and effect. Two studies specifically compared risk of post-ERCP pancreatitis in patients having ERCP for suspected sphincter of Oddi dysfunction with and without sphincter of Oddi manometry and found no detectable independent effect of manometry on risk.[2,13] Patients with suspected choledocholithiasis who are found not to have stone disease are at similarly high risk for post-ERCP pancreatitis, which points out the danger of performing diagnostic ERCP to look for bile duct stones in women with recurrent postcholecystectomy pain, because there is generally a low probability of finding stones in such patients, and a high risk of causing pancreatitis. It is an erroneous and potentially dangerous assumption that merely avoiding sphincter of Oddi manometry significantly reduces risk. Increased use of endoscopic ultrasonography and magnetic resonance cholangiopancreatography (MRCP) determines in advance that such patients do not harbor bile duct stones, and either eliminates the need for conventional ERCP, or allows triage of the patients to ERCP performed with maximal therapeutic benefit (dual sphincter manometry and therapy) and protective measures (pancreatic stents).

A history of previous post-ERCP pancreatitis increases risk substantially (up to 4-fold),[3,4] On the other hand, advanced chronic pancreatitis confers some immunity against ERCP pancreatitis, perhaps because of atrophy and decreased enzymatic activity.[3] Pancreas divisum is a risk factor only if minor papilla cannulation is attempted. Despite many early studies suggesting small bile duct diameter to be a risk factor for pancreatitis, most recent studies have shown no independent influence of duct size on risk; small duct diameter may have been a surrogate marker for sphincter of Oddi dysfunction or patients without true obstructive biliary disease in older studies suggesting higher risk. ERCP for removal of bile duct stones has been found to be relatively safe with respect to pancreatitis rates (usually <3%–4%) in multicenter studies regardless of bile duct diameter.[2] Periampullary diverticula or Billroth II gastrectomy do not seem to influence risk of post-ERCP pancreatitis.[2]

Risk Factors for Post-ERCP Pancreatitis Related to Technique

Technique-related issues have long been recognized to be important in causing post-ERCP pancreatitis. Papillary trauma induced by difficult cannulation has a negative effect that is independent of the number of pancreatic duct contrast injections.[2–10] Importance of contrast injection alone in causing post-ERCP pancreatitis has probably been overemphasized. Pancreatitis occurred after 2.5% of ERCP in 1 study involving no pancreatic duct contrast injection.[3] Acinarization of the pancreas, although undesirable, is probably less important than generally believed and has not been found to be significant in 2 recent studies.[3,4] Risk of pancreatitis is generally similar after diagnostic and therapeutic ERCP.[2–10] Performance of biliary sphincterotomy does not seem to add significant independent risk of pancreatitis to ERCP.[3,4] This observation does not reflect the safety of sphincterotomy, but rather the risk of diagnostic ERCP. Pancreatic sphincterotomy of any kind,[3] including minor papilla sphincterotomy[3,4] has been found to be a significant risk factor for pancreatitis, although the risk of severe pancreatitis has been low (<1%), perhaps because nearly all of these patients had pancreatic drainage via a pancreatic stent.

Risk related to use of precut or access papillotomy is controversial and difficult to sort out from other variables, including difficult cannulation. Use of precut to access bile duct varies widely among endoscopists, from less than 5% to as much as 30% of cases.[14] There are many variations on precut technique: standard needle-knife inserted at the papillary orifice and cutting upwards; needle-knife fistulotomy starting the incision above the papillary orifice and then cutting either up or down; use of a pull-type sphincterotome wedged either in the papillary orifice or transpancreatic precut performed by cutting the pancreatic sphincter intentionally. Any of the access techniques has the potential to lacerate and injure the pancreatic sphincter. Precut techniques have been uniformly associated with a higher risk of pancreatitis by univariate and multivariate analysis in multicenter studies involving endoscopists with varied experience.[2,7] In contrast, many series from tertiary referral centers have found complication rates no different than for standard sphincterotomy, suggesting that risk of precut sphincterotomy is highly operator-dependent.[15] In 1 study, endoscopists performing more than 1 sphincterotomy a week averaged 90% immediate bile duct access after precutting, versus only 50% for lower-volume endoscopists, a success rate that hardly justifies the risk of complications.[2] Comparative studies of precut with standard sphincterotomy are difficult to interpret because indications and settings may be different, with precut preferentially performed in lower-risk situations such as obstructive jaundice, and prominent papillae. In addition, increasing use of pancreatic stents in series from tertiary centers may have neutralized the otherwise higher risk of precut sphincterotomy.[7] Complications of precut sphincterotomy vary with the indication for the procedure, occurring in as many as 30% of patients with sphincter of Oddi dysfunction in older studies without use of pancreatic stents.[2] Paradoxically, in patients with sphincter of Oddi dysfunction, needle-knife sphincterotomy over a pancreatic stent placed early in the procedure has been shown to be substantially safer than conventional pull-type sphincterotomy without a pancreatic stent.[16]

It has been unclear whether increased risk of access papillotomy is because of the technique itself or because of prolonged cannulation attempts, which often precede its use. A meta-analysis of 6 randomized trials comparing precut papillotomy with persistent cannulation provides some insight. These trials included 966 patients assigned to early precut implementation or persistent attempts at standard cannulation.[17] Post-ERCP pancreatitis was significantly less common in patients undergoing precut compared with the group who underwent persistent attempts at cannulation (3% vs 5%). However, the overall rate of complications, including pancreatitis, bleeding, cholangitis, and perforation, did not significantly differ between the 2 groups (5% vs 6%). Limiting the relevance of these studies is the fact that few of these studies included patients with high-risk indications such as sphincter of Oddi dysfunction, or involved use of pancreatic stents, which is now considered fairly standard.

Presence of multiple risk factors for post-ERCP pancreatitis substantially escalates the probability that a patient will develop this complication.[3] The interactive effect of multiple risk factors is reflected in the profile of patients developing severe post-ERCP pancreatitis. In 1 study predating widespread use of pancreatic stents, women with a normal serum bilirubin level had a 5% risk of pancreatitis; with addition of difficult cannulation risk increased to 16%; with further addition of suspected sphincter of Oddi dysfunction (ie, no stone found), the risk increased to 42%.[3] In 2 different studies, nearly all of the patients who developed severe pancreatitis were young to middle-aged women with recurrent abdominal pain, a normal serum bilirubin level, and with no biliary obstructive disease.[3,11] These observations emphasize the importance of tailoring the approach of ERCP to the individual patient.

The effect of endoscopist case volumes and experience on post-ERCP pancreatitis seems to be intuitively obvious, but has been difficult to show. A recent study showed that trainee participation adds independent risk of pancreatitis.[4] In contrast, most multicenter studies have failed to show a significant correlation between endoscopists' ERCP case volumes and pancreatitis rates.[2,3,7] It is possible that none of the participating endoscopists in those studies reached the threshold volume of ERCP above which pancreatitis rates would diminish (perhaps >250–500 cases per year). However, most American endoscopists average fewer than 2 ERCPs per week,[3] and the reported rates of pancreatitis from the highest-volume tertiary referral centers in the United States are often higher than those in private practices. All of these observations suggest that case mix is at least as important as expertise in determining risk of post-ERCP pancreatitis.

Specific Techniques to Reduce Risk of Post-ERCP Pancreatitis

In general, the most atraumatic and efficient method of cannulation is associated with the fewest complications, but the importance of cannulation difficulty in causing pancreatitis has probably been exaggerated. Use of a papillotome or steerable catheter for biliary cannulation has been prospectively compared with a standard catheter in randomized trials.[15] All of these studies showed significantly higher success rates with the sphincterotome or steerable cannula; however, there was no difference in rates of pancreatitis or other complications. Another randomized trial did show significant reduction of pancreatitis risk when a guidewire was used in conjunction with a papillotome, as opposed to a papillotome and conventional contrast injection alone;

the relevance of this study is questionable because few use only a cannula and contrast to access ducts any more.[15]

Using the guidewire as a primary cannulation device is an increasingly used technique, either by leading with the guidewire, or by inserting the cannula or papillotome into the papillary orifice then advancing the guidewire without contrast injection. Guidewire cannulation has been shown to decrease post-ERCP pancreatitis rates in several prospective randomized trials, with rates of 0% to 3% using wire cannulation compared with rates of 4% to 12% using contrast injection. In practice, many advanced endoscopists now use a hybrid of the 2 techniques, using minimal contrast to outline the course of the distal ducts in combination with wire probes. Such a hybrid technique may avoid dissections or passage of the guidewire out a side branch of the pancreatic duct, but has not been formally evaluated.

Thermal injury is believed to play some role in causing pancreatitis after biliary and pancreatic sphincterotomy. Several randomized trials have compared the impact of pure cutting versus blended current, with mixed results but generally lower rates of pancreatitis using the pure cut current.[15] Automated current delivery systems programmed to deliver a specific tissue effect are now widely used. None of the available studies suggests a significant difference in rates of pancreatitis between these units compared with blended current, and it is not yet clear whether automated current delivery systems provide the same benefit for prevention of pancreatitis as do those using pure cutting current.

Pancreatic Stents for Prevention of Post-ERCP Pancreatitis

Pancreatic stent placement is increasingly used as a method to reduce risk of post-ERCP pancreatitis. Such use of pancreatic stents now extends into routine practice, and is increasingly becoming considered standard of care in high-risk circumstances (**Figs. 1** and **2**).[18] Specific situations in which placement of a pancreatic stent has been shown to reduce risk include biliary sphincterotomy for sphincter of Oddi dysfunction, suspected sphincter of Oddi dysfunction with normal manometry, pancreatic sphincterotomy, precut sphincterotomy, balloon dilation of the biliary sphincter, and endoscopic ampullectomy, after pancreatic wire-assisted biliary cannulation, probably after difficult cannulation in general, and even after unselected ERCP in patients with virgin papilla, excluding those with pancreas divisum or cancer (**Table 5**).[18–27]

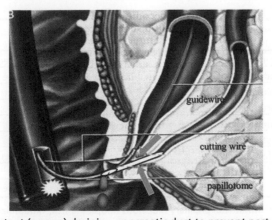

Fig. 1. Pancreatic stent (*arrows*) draining pancreatic duct to prevent post-ERCP pancreatitis.

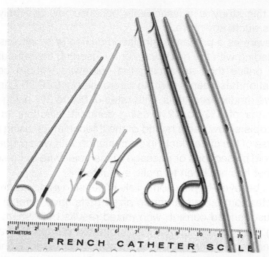

Fig. 2. Wide variety of pancreatic stents used for protection against post-ERCP pancreatitis in normal ducts (5 stents on left half) and therapy for pancreatic strictures (4 stents on right half).

Several meta-analyses have shown that use of pancreatic stents in high-risk patients reduced rates of pancreatitis by about two-thirds, with virtual elimination of severe post-ERCP pancreatitis.[21,26,27] Although effective in high-risk cases, placement of pancreatic stents is usually unnecessary regardless of cannulation difficulty in older, jaundiced patients if they have a pancreatic duct obstructed by cancer. Pancreatic stenting has some limitations as a strategy to reduce risk.[18] Many endoscopists and their assistants are unfamiliar with their placement and may have a substantial failure rate, leaving the patient worse off than if no attempt was made.[23] Small-caliber wires (0.46 mm [0.018 in] or 0.635 mm [0.025 in]) are often optimal for deep insertion into small or tortuous ducts, and ansa pancreaticus (360° α loop), all posing a challenge even for the most experienced endoscopist (**Figs. 3** and **4**). A technique has been described that

Table 5
Pancreatic stents to reduce risk of post-ERCP pancreatitis

Setting	Benefit	Evidence
Biliary sphincterotomy for SOD	Yes	RCT
Suspected SOD with normal manometry	Yes	Retrospective case control
Pancreatic sphincterotomy	Yes	RCT, retrospective case control
Biliary balloon dilation for stone	Trend	Retrospective case control
Precut (access) sphincterotomy	Yes	RCT (abstract)
High risk (eg, difficult cannulation)	Yes/trend	RCT × 2
Pancreatic guidewire-assisted cannulation	Yes	RCT
Pancreatic brush cytology	Trend	Retrospective case control
Endoscopic ampullectomy	Yes/trend	RCT, retrospective case control
All consecutive ERCP, unselected	Yes	RCT × 2
IPMN	No	Retrospective case control

Abbreviations: IPMN, intraductal papillary mucinous neoplasm; RCT, randomized controlled trial; SOD, sphincter of Oddi dysfunction.

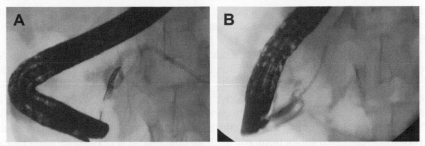

Fig. 3. (*A*) Fluoroscopy showing pancreatic duct with ansa loop (360° loop), with 0.46-mm (0.018-in) wire knuckled just at first turn in duct. (*B*) After delivery of 4-French 2-cm stent in patient from (*A*).

allows universal success at placing stents in difficult anatomy; a small-caliber nitinol-tipped wire can be knuckled inside the main pancreatic duct just beyond the sphincter and allow delivery of a small-caliber short inner flanged stent.[23]

Pancreatic stents may cause complications themselves. Stents may be inadvertently pushed or spontaneously migrate inside the pancreatic duct, especially longer straight stents and those with dual inner flanges. Inward delivery can largely be avoided by use of a single pigtail on the duodenal end, which has a clear visual marker for deployment. Pancreatic stents may cause ductal or parenchymal injury or perforation. Ductal and parenchymal pancreatic injury has been reported to occur in up to 80% of patients with previously normal ducts using conventional 5 French or greater polyethylene stents.[28–31] Although it has been assumed that such injury resolves spontaneously, there have been reports of, and every advanced center has seen cases of, permanent ductal stenosis and relapsing acute and chronic pancreatitis.[31] Strategies to avoid this complication included use of smaller-caliber stents (3 or 4 French), which have been shown to be associated with lower rates of duct injury than conventional polyethylene 5 French stents,[30] and use of stents made of softer materials, which are now widely

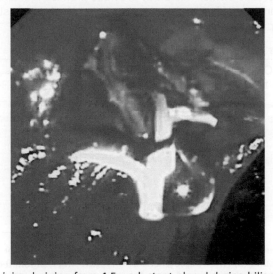

Fig. 4. Pancreatic juice draining from 4-French stent placed during biliary sphincterotomy.

available (**Fig. 5**). Pancreatic stents placed for prevention of post-ERCP pancreatitis should be documented to pass by radiograph or removed within a few weeks.

Balloon dilation of the biliary sphincter has been introduced as an alternative to sphincterotomy for the extraction of bile duct stones, or as an adjunct to biliary sphincterotomy for extraction of large or difficult bile duct stones. Balloon dilation of intact biliary sphincter has been associated with a markedly increased risk of pancreatitis, resulting in 2 deaths in 1 American study,[32] and with a higher risk of pancreatitis by meta-analysis of pooled studies.[33] In general, balloon dilation of the intact biliary sphincter for extraction of bile duct stones is not recommended unless there is a relative contraindication to sphincterotomy such as coagulopathy or need for early anticoagulation, and if it is performed, it should generally be accompanied by placement of a prophylactic pancreatic stent. In contrast, balloon dilation performed after biliary sphincterotomy to facilitate large stone extraction may be relatively safe and may reduce need for excessively large sphincterotomy and its associated risk of perforation or bleeding, such that pancreatic stent placement is optional.[34,35]

Pharmacologic Agents to Prevent Post-ERCP Pancreatitis

Pharmacologic agents have been investigated as potential agents to reduce post-ERCP pancreatitis, with generally mixed or negative results, until recently. Meta-analyses of randomized controlled trials have shown that gabexate (a protease inhibitor) and somatostatin are marginally effective in preventing post-ERCP pancreatitis, but only if given over an extended infusion of up to 12 hours after ERCP, whereas shorter infusions of less than 4 hours are generally ineffective.[15] The lack of cost-effectiveness of prolonged infusions and lack of availability in the United States limits the practicality of these agents. Agents shown not to be effective include interleukin 10, octreotide, corticosteroids, allopurinol, platelet-activating factor inhibitors, heparin, and use of nonionic contrast.[15] More promising agents in pilot studies and a meta-analysis have included nonsteroidal antiinflammatory drugs (NSAIDs), although efficacy in high-risk patients was unclear.[36] A recently published multicenter randomized controlled trial has shown significant reduction of post-ERCP pancreatitis using rectal indomethacin in a high-risk group of patients and procedures, 80% of whom received prophylactic pancreatic stents. This study provides promise that an inexpensive and nontoxic agent can provide further risk reduction beyond pancreatic stenting in a problematic group of patients.[37]

Overall Strategies to Prevent Post-ERCP Pancreatitis

Avoidance of ERCP for marginal indications, especially in patients at higher risk of complications, is the single most effective way to prevent post-ERCP pancreatitis.

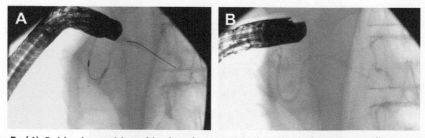

Fig. 5. (*A*) Guidewire positioned in dorsal pancreatic duct through minor papilla in patient with pancreas divisum. (*B*) After deployment of 4-French single-pigtail 9-cm stent made of soft pliable material, conforming to shape of duct, in patient from (*A*).

The risk of complications is often higher and potential benefit of therapy lower in marginally indicated ERCP than for patients with obstructive jaundice. ERCP should generally be avoided outside specialized referral centers when the probability of finding stones or other obstructive disease is low and other methods are available, or situations in which the risk/benefit ratio of conventional diagnostic or biliary therapeutic ERCP is high (such as suspected sphincter of Oddi dysfunction). Alternative imaging techniques such as intraoperative laparoscopic cholangiography, MRCP, and endoscopic ultrasonography are safer alternatives for excluding obstructive biliary disease. Patients who have negative evaluation by these alternative techniques, but who are still suspected to have a pancreatic or biliary cause for recurrent symptoms, are probably best served by referral to a tertiary ERCP center capable of advanced techniques for diagnosis, including endoscopic ultrasonography and advanced therapeutics, including pancreatic endotherapy, for near-certain ability to place pancreatic stents.

Specific ERCP cannulation and sphincterotomy techniques in any given patient are ideally tailored to the risk profile of that individual. In low-risk patients such as elderly patients with obstructive jaundice, manipulation is generally well tolerated, and whatever techniques are effective at gaining bile duct access and drainage are reasonable. In high-risk cases, manipulation should be minimized, and placement of a pancreatic stent considered early in the procedure. Placement of pancreatic stents is recommended in most patients with suspected sphincter dysfunction, history of post-ERCP pancreatitis, difficult cannulation, or before precut sphincterotomy with unclear papillary anatomy or in those with other risk factors. One important strategy in patients at high risk, either because of their profile, or because of events that happen during ERCP, is to access the pancreatic duct with a guidewire and consider stenting the pancreatic duct before rather than after completing intended therapy such as biliary sphincterotomy. This approach avoids the problem of difficulty in accessing the pancreatic duct after distortion of the native anatomy by sphincterotomy or other instrumentation.

It is reasonable to recommend use of rectal indomethacin, when available, to patients judged to be at high risk of post-ERCP pancreatitis. Until further data are available, it is not advisable to forgo placement of pancreatic stents in high-risk cases.

Treatment of post-ERCP pancreatitis is like that for any other cause of acute pancreatitis. Early recognition of impending post-ERCP pancreatitis can be facilitated by checking serum amylase levels or other enzymes within a few hours after the procedure in patients who are at high risk or who have abdominal pain. If serum amylase or lipase level is normal, probability of developing pancreatitis is low and the patient can be considered for same-day discharge if otherwise reasonable. On the other hand, if the pancreatic enzyme levels are significantly increased, and there is clinical suspicion of evolving pancreatitis, premature same-day discharge may be avoided, and preemptive hospitalization for observation, fasting, and vigorous intravenous hydration initiated. If post-ERCP pancreatitis is recognized early in patients without a pancreatic stent, or if there is early dislodgement of a prophylactic stent, there may be a role for immediate repeat ERCP with placement of a salvage stent. Data regarding such an approach are preliminary but encouraging.[38]

POSTSPHINCTEROTOMY HEMORRHAGE

Bleeding observed during sphincterotomy is common but does not represent an adverse outcome to the patient unless there is clinically significant blood loss or change in management. Some degree of bleeding, ranging from oozing to severe bleeding, is seen at the time of sphincterotomy in up to 10% to 30% of cases. Clinically significant hemorrhage is defined in the consensus criteria (see **Table 1**) as clinical evidence of bleeding such as melena or hematemesis, with or without an associated decrease in hemoglobin level, or requirement for secondary intervention such as endoscopy or blood transfusion, and occurs in 0.1% to 2% of sphincterotomies.[2] As for postpolypectomy bleeding, clinical presentation of hemorrhage after sphincterotomy can be delayed up to 10 days after the procedure.[2]

Risk Factors for Hemorrhage After Sphincterotomy

Risk factors for hemorrhage after sphincterotomy have been defined in a large multicenter cohort study, and include any degree of bleeding during the procedure, presence of any coagulopathy or thrombocytopenia (including hemodialysis-associated coagulation disorders), initiation of anticoagulant therapy within 3 days after the procedure, presence of active cholangitis, and relatively low case volume on the part of the endoscopist (defined as performance of not more than 1 sphincterotomy per week).[2] Factors that do not seem to increase risk of bleeding include use of aspirin or NSAIDs, making a longer incision, or extending a previous sphincterotomy (see **Table 4**).[2] The effect of newer antiplatelet agents is unknown.

Methods to Prevent and Treat Hemorrhage After Sphincterotomy

In patients with risk factors such as coagulopathy, postsphincterotomy hemorrhage can be avoided by finding substitute procedures such as balloon dilation of the biliary sphincter. Once sphincterotomy is undertaken, risk can be minimized by correction of any coagulopathies, withholding anticoagulant medications for as many as 3 days afterward, and by use of meticulous endoscopic technique. Prophylactic injection of the sphincterotomy site with epinephrine in patients with coagulopathy has been suggested to possibly reduce risk of delayed bleeding but is of uncertain efficacy. Automated current delivery cautery systems have been shown to reduce risk of immediate bleeding but have not been shown to decrease the incidence of clinically significant hemorrhage, although such complications are increasingly rare.

If significant hemorrhage occurs, either immediately during sphincterotomy, or delayed, it can generally be controlled with endoscopic therapy. First-line treatment includes injection of dilute epinephrine, which can be performed by using a duodenoscope-compatible sclerotherapy needle, but injection can also be performed by inserting an ultratapered cannula or sphincterotome into the cut edges of the sphincterotomy, thereby delivering a submucosal injection. (**Fig. 6**) Balloon tamponade using standard dilating balloons may allow temporary control of bleeding and improve visualization of the bleeding site. Thermal therapy such as bipolar coagulation or placement of clips can follow. Caution should be taken to avoid thermal injury or clip placement over the pancreatic sphincter, especially if the bleeding site is on the right-hand wall of the sphincterotomy incision. Rarely, angiography or surgery is required for refractory bleeding.

PERFORATION

Perforation during ERCP may occur in several forms. First, the bowel wall can be perforated by the endoscope, usually resulting in intraperitoneal perforation; second, extension of a sphincterotomy incision beyond the intramural portion of the bile or pancreatic duct with retroperitoneal leakage, or third, at any location as a result of extramural passage or migration of guidewires or stents. Perforation is now reported in less than 1% of ERCP and sphincterotomies.[2–9] Risk factors for sphincterotomy perforation have been difficult to quantify because of the rarity of perforation. It is probable that bowel perforation is more common in patients with Billroth II or Roux-en-Y anatomy, and sphincterotomy perforation more common after needle-knife

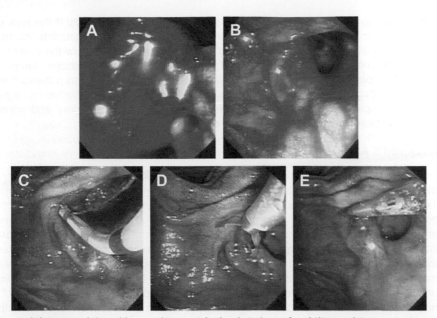

Fig. 6. (*A*) Severe delayed hemorrhage with shock 3 days after biliary sphincterotomy with large balloon dilation and stone extraction in patient with recent carotid artery stent and transient ischemic attacks who was placed on full anticoagulation within 24 hours after ERCP. (*B*) Bleeding site visualized at left apex of sphincterotomy after vigorous lavage and mechanical removal of clot. (*C*) Papillotome used to inject epinephrine submucosally into edge of sphincterotomy by inserting tip of cannula into incision. (*D*) Endoscopic clip placed carefully around left upper edge of sphincterotomy. (*E*) After placement of clip across left apex of sphincterotomy; patulous orifice of previous biliary sphincterotomy is visible behind upper half of the clip.

precut techniques, and in patients with suspected sphincter of Oddi dysfunction, all situations in which control and extent of the required incision are uncertain.

Treatment of post-ERCP perforation varies with the type and severity of the leak and clinical manifestations. Bowel wall perforations are generally treated surgically, although there are increasing applications of endoscopic clipping and use of dedicated endoscopic closure devices to treat larger perforations. Guidewire-related or stent-related perforations can usually be treated endoscopically by providing adequate ductal drainage beyond the leak site.[38–40] Sphincterotomy-related perforation remains the most common and challenging to avoid and treat. Keys to avoiding perforation during sphincterotomy are to limit the length of cutting wire in contact with the tissue and to use stepwise incisions. If perforation is suspected during a sphincterotomy, careful fluoroscopy and injection of a small amount of contrast while pulling the catheter or papillotome through the incision over a guidewire confirm or exclude extravasation and allow proactive treatment. Endoscopic clipping may be attempted to close a definite leak.[40] In most cases, a nasobiliary or nasopancreatic drain should be placed (depending on the sphincter cut). Another approach to biliary sphincterotomy is to place a fully covered removable self-expanding metallic stent to drain the bile duct and occlude the leak. Regardless of endoscopic therapy, the patient is generally treated with nasogastric suction, intravenous antibiotics, strict fasting, surgical consultation, and in-hospital observation. Once a perforation of any kind is suspected, a computed tomography scan of the abdomen should be obtained to assess for contrast leakage and any retroperitoneal or intraperitoneal air (**Fig. 7**). If the leak is sizable and continuing as suggested by ongoing contrast extravasation, or the patient's clinical condition deteriorates, prompt drainage via surgery or the percutaneous route is advisable. The importance of early recognition and endoscopic drainage of suspected perforations is supported by the observation that nearly all patients with immediate recognition and endoscopic drainage did well with conservative management, in comparison with poor outcomes, including need for surgery and some mortality, in patients with delayed recognition.[39,40]

CHOLANGITIS AND CHOLECYSTITIS

Cholangitis (ascending bile duct infection) and cholecystitis (gallbladder infection) are potential complications or sequelae of ERCP or sphincterotomy, and of biliary stents, whether plastic or metallic. Risk factors for cholangitis after ERCP and sphincterotomy consist primarily of failed or incomplete biliary drainage[2–9] and use of combined percutaneous-endoscopic procedures.[2] Other risk factors may include jaundice, especially if caused by malignancy, and operator inexperience.[2] Several studies have shown that prophylactic antibiotics can reduce the rate of bacteremia, but few studies have shown a reduction in clinical sepsis after ERCP, and a meta-analysis concluded that there was no clinical benefit to routine administration of antibiotics.[41] Thus the principal recommendation regarding prevention and treatment of cholangitis is obtaining successful and complete biliary drainage. Once recognized, cholecystitis can be managed conservatively, by surgery, by percutaneous drainage, and increasingly by transpapillary gallbladder drainage at ERCP.

LONG-TERM CONSEQUENCES OF SPHINCTEROTOMY

Recent studies have shown that if the gallbladder is left intact after sphincterotomy, both early and late cholecystitis may occur. Both cholecystitis and recurrent bile duct stones are more common if the gallbladder left in situ contains stones. There is increasing concern about potential long-term sequelae of various components of endoscopic therapy, including endoscopic biliary and pancreatic sphincterotomy. These sequelae include recurrent stone formation, possibly resulting from sphincterotomy stenosis, or bacterobilia caused by duodenal-biliary reflux, or sine-materia cholangitis. Recurrent stones and other biliary problems may occur in from 6% to 24% of patients undergoing long-term follow-up. Recurrent pancreatitis, presumably

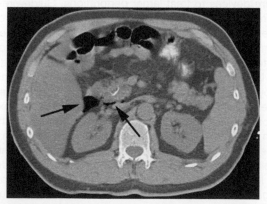

Fig. 7. Retroperitoneal air (*arrows*) after endoscopic ampullectomy for ampullary adenoma complicated by immediate perforation, which was successfully closed with endoscopic clips.

caused by thermal injury to the pancreatic sphincter, may occur after biliary sphincterotomy. The long-term effects of pancreatic sphincterotomy, which is increasingly performed in patients with and without chronic pancreatitis, are largely unknown.

ENDOSCOPISTS' EXPERIENCE AND COMPLICATIONS OF ERCP

The effect of endoscopic expertise on outcomes of ERCP is intuitively obvious but difficult to evaluate scientifically. Simple comparisons of complication rates of ERCP between centers are misleading, because the reporting methodology, case mix, intent of the procedure, and success rates at achieving biliary and pancreatic duct access vary widely. Several studies have evaluated endoscopist-related factors in complications of ERCP. Lower ERCP case volume, defined variably, has been associated with higher overall complications by univariate and multivariate analysis in all studies that have evaluated that risk factor. In 1 study, endoscopists who performed more than 1 sphincterotomy per week had significantly lower rates of overall complications (8% vs 11%), but substantially lower rates of severe complications (0.9% vs 2.3%)[2]; in a multivariate model using only information available before ERCP, lower procedure volume was 1 of only 3 variables that predicted complications of sphincterotomy.[2] Lower case volume was significantly associated with higher rates of hemorrhage after sphincterotomy in 2 studies.[2,7] On the other hand, lower ERCP case volume has not consistently been found to correlate with rates of post-ERCP pancreatitis, suggesting the importance of case mix in determining this complication.

In 1 multicenter study, endoscopists were considered high volume if they performed more than 50 procedures a year. In that study, endoscopists with high case volume had better diagnostic and therapeutic success (86.9% vs 80.3%) with fewer complications (10.2% vs 13.6%) than endoscopists with lower case volume.[42] In an older but similar study from Italy, complications were substantially higher (7.1% vs 2.0%) after ERCP performed in centers with low volumes (<200/y) compared with high-volume centers.[7] In an American multicenter study, endoscopists who carried out less than 1 sphincterotomy per week had higher complication rates compared with their peers who performed higher volumes of sphincterotomies each week.[2] These and other studies[43,44] support the concept that a lower case volume affects outcomes adversely. In contrast, another recent large multicenter study of assessment of risk factors for ERCP complications from Great Britain found no difference in overall complications between endoscopists of differing case loads or hospital type.[9] The only difference found was a decrease in the risk of post-ERCP pancreatitis when the procedure was performed at a university hospital compared with a district hospital, a finding that has been interpreted to perhaps reflect the better support staff and environment available at university hospitals.

The available data probably underestimate the influence of operator experience on outcomes of ERCP, for many reasons. First, high-volume endoscopists generally attempt higher-risk and more challenging cases, but despite that also have higher success rates at duct access. In 1 study, endoscopists averaging more than 100 ERCP cases per year had 96.5% success at bile duct access compared with 91.5% for lower-volume endoscopists.[3] In 2 other multicenter studies, rates for failure and complications of ERCP by higher-volume endoscopists were significantly lower than those of lesser-volume endoscopists.[2,7] Failure to complete ERCP may have as much negative impact on patients as complications in terms of cost, need for further interventions, and extension of hospital stay.

The minimum volume of cases required to maintain optimal proficiency at ERCP is unknown, but is probably in excess of 50 to 100 cases per year for routine biliary therapy, and 200 to 250 cases per year for advanced pancreatic techniques. A few endoscopists in the United States achieve such volumes of ERCP. The data suggest that outcomes are optimal if fewer endoscopists perform more ERCP. It is not feasible or palatable to suggest that all ERCP be performed at advanced centers. Rather, adequate training and ongoing case volume should be a prerequisite for performing ERCP in practice. Fourth-year advanced endoscopy fellowships allow the best milieu for acquisition of competency at ERCP and related procedures. A registry of advanced endoscopy fellowships is maintained by the American Society for Gastrointestinal Endoscopy (http://www.asge.org).

Once in practice, establishing and maintaining expertise at ERCP becomes a great challenge. One solution is for larger groups to concentrate all their ERCP to a few dedicated individuals rather than dilute the procedure throughout their practice. For smaller groups who are unable to sustain adequate volumes, another possibility is to contract their ERCP work out to more experienced individuals or refer to advanced centers. Regardless of the context or practice environment, endoscopists who perform limited amounts of complex ERCP should be amenable to prompt referral to a specialized center of potentially complex cases including difficult biliary problems, all pancreatic therapeutics, and most cases of suspected sphincter of Oddi dysfunction. The key is for each endoscopist to find the optimal balance between risk and benefit for the individual patient and their own individual expertise and experience.

REFERENCES

1. Cotton PB, Lehman G, Vennes JA, et al. Endoscopic sphincterotomy complications and their management: an attempt at consensus. Gastrointest Endosc 1991;37: 383–91.
2. Freeman ML, Nelson DB, Sherman S, et al. Complications of endoscopic biliary sphincterotomy. N Engl J Med 1996;335:909–18.
3. Freeman ML, DiSario JA, Nelson DB, et al. Risk factors for post-ERCP pancreatitis: a prospective, multicenter study. Gastrointest Endosc 2001;54:425–34.
4. Cheng CL, Sherman S, Watkins JL, et al. Risk factors for post-ERCP pancreatitis: a prospective multicenter study. Am J Gastroenterol 2006;101:139–47.
5. Vandervoort J, Soetikno RM, Tham TC, et al. Risk factors for complications after performance of ERCP. Gastrointest Endosc 2002;56:652–6.
6. Masci E, Toti G, Mariani A, et al. Complications of diagnostic and therapeutic ERCP: a prospective multicenter study. Am J Gastroenterol 2001;96:417–23.
7. Loperfido S, Angelini G, Benedetti G, et al. Major early complications from diagnostic and therapeutic ERCP: a prospective multicenter study. Gastrointest Endosc 1998;48:1–10.
8. Wang P, Li ZS, Liu F, et al. Risk factors for ERCP-related complications: a prospective multicenter study. Am J Gastroenterol 2009;104:31–40.
9. Williams EJ, Taylor S, Fairclough P, et al. Risk factors for complication following ERCP: results of a large-scale, prospective multicenter study. Endoscopy 2007;9: 793–802.
10. Masci E, Mariani A, Curioni S, et al. Risk factors for pancreatitis following endoscopic retrograde cholangiopancreatography: a meta-analysis. Endoscopy 2003; 35:830–4.
11. Trap R, Adamsen S, Hart-Hansen O, et al. Severe and fatal complications after diagnostic and therapeutic ERCP: a prospective series of claims to insurance covering public hospitals. Endoscopy 1999;31:125–30.

12. Cennamo V, Fuccio L, Rocco M, et al. Can a wire-guided cannulation technique increase bile duct cannulation rate and prevent post-ERCP pancreatitis?: A meta-analysis of randomized controlled trials. Am J Gastroenterol 2009;104:2343–50.
13. Singh P, Gurudu SR, Davidoff S, et al. Sphincter of Oddi manometry does not predispose to post-ERCP acute pancreatitis. Gastrointest Endosc 2004;59: 499–505.
14. Andriulli A, Loperfido S, Napolitano G, et al. Incidence rates of post-ERCP complications: a systematic survey of prospective studies. Am J Gastroenterol 2007;102:1781–8.
15. Freeman ML, Guda NL. Cannulation techniques for ERCP: a review of reported techniques. Gastrointest Endosc 2005;61:112–25.
16. Fogel EL, Eversman D, Jamidar P, et al. Sphincter of Oddi dysfunction: pancreaticobiliary sphincterotomy with pancreatic stent placement has a lower rate of pancreatitis than biliary sphincterotomy alone. Endoscopy 2002;34:280–5.
17. Cennamo V, Fuccio L, Zagari RM, et al. Can early precut implementation reduce endoscopic retrograde cholangiopancreatography-related complication risk? Meta-analysis of randomized controlled trials. Endoscopy 2010;42:381.
18. Freeman ML. Pancreatic stents for prevention of post-ERCP pancreatitis: for everyday practice or for experts only? Gastrointest Endosc 2010;71:940–4.
19. Tarnasky P, Palesch Y, Cunningham J, et al. Pancreatic stenting prevents pancreatitis after biliary sphincterotomy in patients with sphincter of Oddi dysfunction. Gastroenterology 1998;115:1518–24.
20. Fazel A, Quadri A, Catalano MF, et al. Does a pancreatic duct stent prevent post-ERCP pancreatitis? A prospective randomized study. Gastrointest Endosc 2003; 57:291–4.
21. Singh P, Das A, Isenberg G, et al. Does prophylactic pancreatic stent placement reduce the risk of post-ERCP acute pancreatitis? A meta-analysis of controlled trials. Gastrointest Endosc 2004;60:544–50.
22. Harewood GC, Pochron NL, Gostout CJ. Prospective, randomized, controlled trial of prophylactic pancreatic stent placement for endoscopic snare excision of the duodenal ampulla. Gastrointest Endosc 2005;62:367–70.
23. Freeman ML, Overby CS, Qi DF. Pancreatic stent insertion: consequences of failure, and results of a modified technique to maximize success. Gastrointest Endosc 2004;59:8–14.
24. Sofuni A, Maguchi H, Mukai T, et al. Endoscopic pancreatic duct stents reduce the incidence of post-endoscopic retrograde cholangiopancreatography pancreatitis in high-risk patients. Clin Gastroenterol Hepatol 2011;9:851–8.
25. Freeman ML. Pancreatic stents for prevention of post-endoscopic retrograde cholangiopancreatography pancreatitis. Clin Gastroenterol Hepatol 2007;5: 1354–65.
26. Choudhary A, Bechtold ML, Arif M, et al. Pancreatic stents for prophylaxis against post-ERCP pancreatitis: a meta-analysis and systematic review. Gastrointest Endosc 2011;73:275–82.
27. Mazaki T, Masuda H, Takayama T. Prophylactic pancreatic stent placement and post-ERCP pancreatitis: a systematic review and meta-analysis. Endoscopy 2010;42:842–53.
28. Smith MT, Sherman S, Ikenberry SO, et al. Alterations in pancreatic ductal morphology following polyethylene pancreatic stent therapy. Gastrointest Endosc 1996;44:268–75.
29. Kozarek RA. Pancreatic stents can induce ductal changes consistent with chronic pancreatitis. Gastrointest Endosc 1990;36:93–5.

30. Rashdan A, Fogel EL, McHenry L Jr, et al. Improved stent characteristics for prophylaxis of post-ERCP pancreatitis. Clin Gastroenterol Hepatol 2004;2:322–9.
31. Bakman YG, Safdar K, Freeman ML. Pancreatic stent-induced ductal injury: clinical implications and outcomes of endoscopic therapy. Endoscopy 2009;41: 1095–8.
32. Disario JA, Freeman ML, Bjorkman DJ, et al. Endoscopic balloon dilation compared with sphincterotomy for extraction of bile duct stones. Gastroenterology 2004;127:1291–9.
33. Baron TH, Harewood GC. Endoscopic balloon dilation of the biliary sphincter compared to endoscopic biliary sphincterotomy for removal of common bile duct stones during ERCP: a metaanalysis of randomized, controlled trials. Am J Gastroenterol 2004;99:1455–60.
34. Attam R, Freeman ML. Endoscopic papillary large balloon dilation for large common bile duct stones. J Hepatobiliary Pancreat Surg 2009;16:618–23.
35. Freeman ML, Guda NM. Prevention of post-ERCP pancreatitis: a comprehensive review. Gastrointest Endosc 2004;59:845–64.
36. Elmunzer BJ, Waljee AK, Elta GH, et al. A meta-analysis of rectal NSAIDs in the prevention of post-ERCP pancreatitis. Gut 2008;57:1262–7.
37. Elmunzer BJ, Scheiman JM, Lehman GA, et al. A randomized trial of rectal indomethacin to prevent post-ERCP pancreatitis. N Engl J Med 2012;366:1414–22.
38. Madacsy L, Kurucsai G, Joo I, et al. ERCP and insertion of a small-caliber pancreatic stent to prevent the evolution of severe post-ERCP pancreatitis: a case-controlled series. Surg Endosc 2009;23:1887–93.
39. Enns R, Eloubeidi MA, Mergener K. ERCP-related perforations: risk factors and management. Endoscopy 2002;34:293–8.
40. Howard TJ, Tan T, Lehman GA, et al. Classification and management of perforations complicating endoscopic sphincterotomy. Surgery 1999;126(4):658–63.
41. Harris A, Chan AC, Torres-Viera C, et al. Meta-analysis of antibiotic prophylaxis in endoscopic retrograde cholangiopancreatography (ERCP). Endoscopy 1999;9: 718–24.
42. Kapral C, Duller C, Wewalka F, et al. Case volume and outcome of endoscopic retrograde cholangiopancreatography: results of a nationwide Austrian benchmarking project. Endoscopy 2008;40:625–31.
43. Masci E, Minoli G, Rossi M, et al. Prospective multicenter quality assessment of endotherapy of biliary stones: does center volume matter? Endoscopy 2007;39: 1076–81.
44. Guda NM, Freeman ML. How many ERCPs should you do to not harm your patients? Endoscopy 2008;40:675–6.

Endoscopic Retrograde Cholangiopancreatography
Maximizing Benefits and Minimizing Risks

Peter B. Cotton, MD, FRCS, FRCP

KEYWORDS

- Endoscopic retrograde cholangiopancreatography • Pancreatic disease
- Risk factors for adverse events • Biliary system access

KEY POINTS

- Endoscopic retrograde cholangiopancreatography (ERCP) has become enormously popular throughout the world because of its proven value in the management of patients with known and suspected biliary and pancreatic disease.
- Like all invasive interventions, the results of ERCP are operator dependent, and there are significant risks.
- Adverse events can occur in the best of hands, but are more likely when procedures are performed by endoscopists with inadequate training and experience.
- Quality has been described as "doing the right thing, and doing it right." The best outcomes should occur when procedures are done for the best reasons, using optimal techniques in an ideal environment, by the best team, conscious of the risks and the best ways to minimize them.

Endoscopic retrograde cholangiopancreatography (ERCP) has become enormously popular throughout the world because of its proven value in the management of patients with known and suspected biliary and pancreatic disease. Like all invasive interventions, the results of ERCP are operator dependent, and there are significant risks. Adverse events can occur in the best of hands, but are more likely when procedures are performed by endoscopists with inadequate training and experience. Practitioners (and their professional organizations), payors, and patients (and plaintiffs) should all be interested in ensuring the highest possible benefit/risk ratios in ERCP practice. Quality has been described as "doing the right thing, and doing it right." The best outcomes should occur when procedures are done for the best reasons, using optimal techniques in an ideal environment and a well-trained team, conscious of the risks and the ways to minimize them. These intertwining elements are discussed sequentially in this article.

Department of Digestive Disease Center, Medical University of South Carolina, 25 Courtenay Drive, ART 7100A, MSC 290, Charleston, SC 29425 2900, USA
E-mail address: cottonp@musc.edu

Gastrointest Endoscopy Clin N Am 22 (2012) 587–599
doi:10.1016/j.giec.2012.05.002
1052-5157/12/$ – see front matter © 2012 Elsevier Inc. All rights reserved.

DOING THE RIGHT THING

An ERCP procedure, like any other, may be recommended for many reasons: to make or refine a diagnosis, to assess the status of a known disease (surveillance), to screen for disease, to take target specimens, to provide treatment, or combinations of the above. For any one patient, the overall goal of the procedure is framed by the specific clinical context, which can be described by many elements, including symptoms (eg, jaundice or pain), findings (eg, laboratory tests and images), prior surgery (eg, cholecystectomy), comorbidities, and other factors increasing risk or complexity.

Indications

Professional societies such as the American Society for Gastrointestinal Endoscopy (ASGE) have produced lists of approved indications (**Box 1**), and include adherence to them as key metrics of procedural quality.[1,2]

Review of this list of ASGE indications reveals its obvious shortcomings. The legitimacy of many of the indications (eg, A through E) depends entirely on the extent of the prior workup, and the level of diagnostic suspicion. Item B is so broad as to be virtually meaningless. F says that sphincter of Oddi manometry is an approved indication, but clearly that would depend entirely on the clinical context. Indication K begs the

---

Box 1
Indications for ERCP

A. Jaundice thought to be the result of biliary obstruction

B. Clinical and biochemical or imaging data suggestive of pancreatic or biliary tract disease

C. Signs or symptoms suggesting pancreatic malignancy when direct imaging results are equivocal or normal

D. Pancreatitis of unknown etiology

E. Preoperative evaluation of chronic pancreatitis or pancreatic pseudocyst

F. Sphincter of Oddi manometry

G. Endoscopic sphincterotomy

   1. Choledocholithiasis

   2. Papillary stenosis or sphincter of Oddi dysfunction causing disability

   3. Facilitate biliary stent placement or balloon dilatation

   4. Sump syndrome

   5. Choledochocele

   6. Ampullary carcinoma in poor surgical candidates

   7. Access to pancreatic duct

H. Stent placement across benign or malignant strictures, fistulae, postoperative bile leak, or large common bile duct stones

I. Balloon dilatation of ductal strictures

J. Nasobiliary drain placement

K. Pseudocyst drainage in appropriate cases

L. Tissue sampling from pancreatic or bile ducts

M. Pancreatic therapeutics

question, by stating "pseudocyst drainage in appropriate cases." M states that "pancreatic therapeutics" is an indication, but surely also only in "appropriate cases."

Furthermore, ERCP is not performed in a technical vacuum. There is now a plethora of relevant diagnostic procedures such as magnetic resonance cholangiopancreatography and endoscopic ultrasonography, which may obviate ERCP or better focus its application. In addition, surgery has become much safer over the years, and may well provide more definitive treatment in some contexts, for example, chronic pancreatitis. The report from the National Institutes of Health (NIH) "state of the science" conference on ERCP made many comments on alternative approaches and quality issues.[3]

Careful consideration of these alternatives (and the level of expertise available locally) is needed before concluding that ERCP Is the legitimate procedure of choice in the precise patient and clinical context. This aspect is often the issue in lawsuits when it is argued that something less invasive than ERCP might have been preferred. These issues and the evidence behind them are discussed in articles elsewhere in this issue that deal with individual clinical contexts.

Better ways to document the reasons for doing a procedure (the indication)
Endoscopy reports traditionally include the indication for the procedure. An important practical issue is how to express this succinctly and meaningfully, especially in electronic reporting systems, which demand structured data sets. For the reasons argued above, simply ticking a box of ASGE-approved indications is insufficient. It is preferable to define and document all of the individual elements that go into making a procedural recommendation in a matrix:

- Overall goal
- Planned procedures (strategy)
- Symptoms
- Known and suspected diseases
- Recent laboratory tests and images
- Prior surgeries
- Prior interventions (eg, prior stents)
- Comorbidities and risk factors.

This matrix would be comprehensive, allow some detailed research analysis, and might help in medicolegal conflicts, whereby the need for the (complicated) procedure is often at issue. The data entered could also easily be mapped to any other proposed list, because it will contain all of the elements. However, these lists would be long, and most endoscopists will argue that the details should already be available in their preprocedure clinical report (assuming that there is one). A simpler approach is to note the general clinical context, as is used in the ERCP Quality Network (**Box 2**).[4]

A similar approach is taken in the latest iteration of the Minimal Standard Terminology (MST 3.0), where indications are replaced by "reasons for" procedures.[5] The endoscopist has simply to pick a suspected (or known) diagnosis, and add whether the goal is to make or refine a diagnosis, perform therapy, take specimens, or do surveillance or screening.

DOING IT RIGHT

Patients and their caregivers expect that their procedures will be performed for the right reasons but also expeditiously, skillfully, successfully, safely, and comfortably. These expectations can be expanded to make a list of desirable characteristics for all types of endoscopic procedures.

Box 2
Procedural contexts in the ERCP Quality Network

- Obstructive jaundice
- Abnormal liver tests
- Stone, known or probable
- Pancreatitis, acute, active
- Pancreatitis, idiopathic, recurrent
- Pancreatitis, chronic
- Pancreatic pseudocyst/leak
- Pain—chronic, ?cause
- Pain—intermittent, eg, postcholecystectomy (includes? sphincter of Oddi dysfunction)
- Biliary postsurgical problem (leak, stricture)
- Stent service, biliary (ie, change or remove)
- Stent service, pancreatic (ie, change or remove)
- Clarify biliary image findings
- Clarify pancreatic image findings
- Tumor ablation
- Other context

- Competent endoscopist
- Appropriate environment, support team, and behavior
- Adequate information
- Strategies to minimize risk, including preprocedure evaluation and monitoring
- Appropriate use of medications, including sedation/analgesia
- Correct selection of equipment, well maintained and processed
- Complete survey of the target organ(s)
- Recognition of all abnormalities, and photodocumentation
- Appropriate tissue sampling
- Application of indicated therapy
- Reasonable duration of procedure and any fluoroscopy
- Smooth recovery, explanation, and discharge
- Recognizing, and managing, adverse events
- Clear explanations, recommendations, and follow-up plans
- Integrated pathology results and necessary communications
- Complete documentation.

Many organizations and groups have explored these quality issues and their metrics.[1,6–9] Most attention has been directed toward the contentious and complex issue of endoscopist competence.

What is a Competent Endoscopist?

In discussing competence it is important to appreciate that ERCP is not a single procedure, but simply describes a method for accessing the biliary system and pancreas through the mouth, for diagnostic and therapeutic interventions. There are many clinical situations for which it may be appropriate, and many techniques and therapies that can be applied. More than 10 years ago, Schutz and Abbot[10] introduced a grading system for "degrees of difficulty," which was intended to help plan ERCP training programs and to define levels of practice. It has been in widespread use subsequently, and divides ERCP practice into 3 levels. Grade 1, or standard, cases are those commonly needed in the community, and include management of bile duct stones (<10 mm), malignant biliary strictures below the hilum, and postoperative biliary leaks. Grade 2 (advanced) includes more complex cases, including: diagnostic ERCP after Billroth II gastrectomy; management of larger stones, benign biliary strictures, and hilar tumors; and minor papilla cannulation. Grade 3 are those cases usually restricted to tertiary centers, including suspected sphincter of Oddi dysfunction, therapeutics after surgical biliary diversion, intrahepatic stones, and all pancreatic therapies. ERCP has changed over the years, and an ASGE working party recently revised the grading system.[11]

These complexity-grading systems have obvious implications for training and practice. Most fellowship programs in the United States attempt only to bring trainees to competence in basic-level procedures (if they offer ERCP training at all). The early assumption that endoscopists might become competent in basic ERCP after being involved in 100 procedures was shown to be far short of the mark by a seminal study from Jowell and colleagues.[12] Their fellows at Duke University were barely achieving 80% competence in basic skills after 180 to 200 cases. Several countries have used this number subsequently as a threshold for competence assessment, but Australia has gone further, and now requires completion of 200 procedures without assistance.[13] Substantially more training, for instance 300 more cases, is required to approach competence in more complex cases, and some will eventually become true experts after years of high-volume practice.

Who Will Do Your ERCP?

Highly skilled ERCPists have technical success rates approaching 100% for most procedures, at least those at basic grade 1. However, not all patients can be managed by these experts. The issue then is how to determine who decides what constitutes acceptable performance, and how patients know who to consult, or maybe who to avoid. Would you let your recent trainee loose on your family? Would you yourself submit to an 80% to 85% ERCPist? This level of performance would be acceptable, perhaps life-saving, in an urgent and remote situation, but certainly not for an elective procedure when experts are available nearby. Those of us working in gastroenterology usually have a reasonably good idea who to refer ERCP cases to (or to consult oneself), based on local reputation and track record. If in doubt, it is often wise to ask the nursing staff! But how is the average patient to know who is competent? ERCP is different from other endoscopies in that it is virtually always performed in hospitals, which have systems for assessing competence and granting privileges. One might assume that hospitals grant privileges only after careful review of relevant data, such as the nature and extent of training, subsequent practice (if any), continuing education, and some performance statistics, as recommended by ASGE and other organizations.[14] However, the author suspects that the process is often more cursory, consisting only of a letter from the training institution. Those writing such letters are smart enough usually simply to confirm that training has been given, not that competence has been achieved. Both training directors and hospitals have been sued for allegedly supporting privileges for endoscopists who have had bad outcomes. It is noteworthy that privileges for ERCP are usually all or none. It would be logical to use the complexity-grading system to allocate levels of privilege.

Proof of competence can only be derived from documentation of performance. There is no substitute for collecting relevant data. Trainees in most countries are now expected to maintain logbooks of their procedural activity during training, and the ASGE and other authorities have recommended that endoscopists should collect data prospectively on their endoscopic practice and performance with "report cards."[15,16]

Report cards and benchmarking performance

Endoscopists cannot be expected to populate their report cards with all of the data elements that have been listed in various well-meaning publications. Items should be selected based on ease of data collection, and by assumed relative importance. Some items are easily recorded, and already appear in most procedure reports (eg, anatomic extent, duration, diagnosis, treatments, immediate adverse events). Other items are more subjective (eg, lesion interpretation), or more difficult to record (eg, delayed events, endoscopist-specific patient satisfaction). Some items would appear to be more important markers of quality than others. For ERCP, selective cannulation and stone extraction rates are obvious key parameters.[2,9]

Once several practitioners agree to share their data, they can compare their practices and levels of performance with those of their peers and "competitors," which requires organization as well as motivation.

With the support of Olympus America, the author's group set up a pilot project, the ERCP Quality Network, to test the practicality and acceptability of collecting and comparing data on the practice and quality of ERCP procedures by individual endoscopists.[4] Baseline information included the experience and practice environment of the endoscopists. Data on each procedure are loaded onto a secure Web site. The data points include the clinical context (indications), complexity grade, American Society of Anesthesiologists (ASA) grade, sedation/anesthesia, admission policy, scope and fluoroscopy times, and success rates for individual technical procedures such as deep biliary cannulation, sphincterotomy, stenting, and adverse events. There are no patient identifiers. The data are analyzed automatically, and results posted immediately on the Web site. Contributors can view a summary of their own performance (report card), and compare it with that of all other contributors to the system (benchmarking), not identified by name. To date, more than 150 ERCPists from several countries have entered data on more than 25,000 cases. The variation in individual biliary cannulation rates is shown in **Fig. 1**.

The Quality Network project shows that data can be collected, shared, and compared by a small number of enthusiastic volunteers, with some commercial support. What might motivate the main body of practitioners? Ultimately, informed consumers will drive this agenda. Practitioners with poor outcomes, or those who choose not to provide data, will be disadvantaged. Keeping a report card will provide a competitive

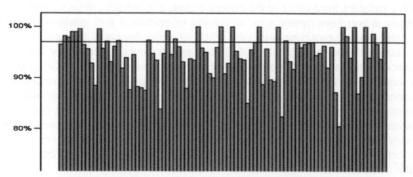

Fig. 1. Average biliary cannulation rates by individual endoscopists in the ERCP Quality Network.

advantage, as intelligent patients will increasingly wish to have greater control over their treatments. It should also provide some medicolegal protection, and will eventually be a crucial tool in the evolving use of "pay for performance" in the United States. The increasing use of electronic endoscopy reporting systems will make this process easy, even automatic.

Is ongoing volume important?

It is logical to assume that anyone offering ERCP should be doing it on a regular basis, to maintain skills and, hopefully, to continue to improve. Several studies have shown that more is better,[8,17–21] but none have data sufficient to define a minimum number (mainly because the lower-volume practitioners do not publish their results). The number probably varies according to the extent of prior practice and the volume of the institution. The British Society of Gastroenterology (BSG) has recommended a minimum of 75 per year.[22] A recent survey of ERCP practice among more than 1000 ASGE members showed that 40% were doing less than 50 per year,[23] data that stimulated an editorial entitled "Are low-volume ERCPists a problem in USA?"[24]

Teamwork and environment

As ERCP has become almost completely therapeutic its needs have become more complex, and increasingly resemble those of traditional surgery, that is, purpose-designed rooms with high-quality fluoroscopy, complex equipment, sterility (where possible), anesthesia, and specially trained staff. Doing complex procedures on uncomfortable patients in unfamiliar territory with untrained staff is a recipe for failure and potential disaster, and this is more likely to be the case in centers with low volumes of ERCP. Recognizing this issue, the BSG has suggested that ERCP should only be performed in centers with more than 200 cases per year.[22] In such light it is striking that a recent survey suggests that about half of all hospitals offering ERCP in the United States do less than 50 per year.[25]

What are the Benefits of ERCP?

Doing the right thing and doing it right should maximize the benefit from an individual procedure, but measuring that benefit is difficult.[7] It can be determined only if the goal is defined beforehand, and the metrics of benefit vary according to the stated goal. Technical success (eg, removal of a stone or placement of a stent) is easy to assess immediately. However, clinical success is a much more elusive and potentially subjective matter, not least because of the time scales involved. Whether sphincterotomy helps a patient with suspected sphincter of Oddi dysfunction, or stenting helps someone with a pancreatic stricture, cannot be assessed until many months have passed. Even if things seem to go well initially, relapse is not unusual. Furthermore, the degree of perceived benefit may be shaded by the level of expectation. It is known that current stents placed for malignant biliary strictures will clog eventually, so that benefit for only a few months is what is hoped for. However, a permanently patent stent would obviously be more beneficial.

We should never forget that the value of ERCP treatments remains controversial in many contexts because we simply do not have enough outcomes data from objective prospective long-term clinical studies. The evidence available in specific contexts is discussed in the other articles in this issue. We should be modest (and honest) when recommending ERCP as the best approach for an individual patient.

What are the Risks of ERCP?

Patients and practitioners expect that their endoscopy procedures will go smoothly and according to plan. There are several reasons why they may be disappointed.

The procedure may fail technically (eg, incomplete colonoscopy or failed biliary cannulation). It may appear to be successful technically but turn out to be clinically unhelpful (eg, a diagnosis missed or an unsuccessful treatment), or there may be an early relapse (eg, stent dysfunction). In addition, some patients and relatives may be disappointed by discourtesy and poor communications, even when everything otherwise works well.

The most feared negative outcome is when something "goes wrong" and the patient suffers a "complication." This term has unfortunate medicolegal connotations, and is perhaps better avoided. Describing these deviations from the plan as "unplanned events" fits nicely with the principles of informed consent, but the term "adverse events" is now in common parlance.

Adverse events can happen before the endoscope is introduced (eg, a reaction to prophylactic antibiotics or bowel-cleansing preparation), during the procedure (eg, hypoxia), immediately afterward (eg, pain due to perforation), a few hours later (eg, pancreatitis after ERCP), or can be delayed for several days or weeks (eg, aspiration pneumonia or delayed bleeding). Some events (eg, viral transmission) may be so far delayed that the connection is difficult to make, or is missed completely.

Defining adverse events

There is a substantial literature describing individual adverse events, and many large collected series.[26,27] A key issue is the need for a standardized nomenclature and agreed definitions for adverse events. For example, what is meant by "hypoxia," or "bleeding," or "infection"? At what level do they become significant enough to be "counted"? Another problem is how to classify and report delayed events, which may or may not be attributable to the procedure. This lack of standardization has many consequences. It hampers the comparison of data from different research and quality-improvement studies. It makes individual studies suspect, because practitioners may not be consistent with their own perceptions and definitions. Furthermore, it makes it impossible to compare endoscopic outcomes with those from other disciplines such as surgery. The need for standardized nomenclature has come into closer focus recently with the increasing use of electronic report writers, which demand a lexicon.

Some attempts were made years ago to address this problem,[28,29] and some 20-year-old definitions for adverse events in ERCP[30] have been widely used, but there has not been consensus across the whole range of endoscopic procedures. The ASGE Quality Task Force convened a workshop in September 2008 to explore the current situation and to make recommendations. Invitations were issued to representatives from the ASGE, the American College of Gastroenterology, and the Society of American Gastrointestinal and Endoscopic Surgeons, and also to those familiar with related lexicons, such as NSQIP (Surgery), HI-IQ (Radiology), NIH, CCTAE (National Cancer Institute), Snomed Clinical Terminology, and the MST. The working party made several recommendations.[31]

Recommendations of the ASGE Working Party on Adverse Events

1. Definitions and severity criteria should be generic across the different endoscopic procedures, although certain events will occur only after some of them (eg, cholangitis after ERCP).
2. An adverse event is one that prevents completion of the planned procedure, and/or results in admission to hospital, or prolongation of existing hospital stay, or (for management of the event) another procedure (one needing sedation/anesthesia), or consultation with another specialty.
3. Timing. Events should be recorded as happening preprocedure, intraprocedure (from entering the preparation area through leaving the endoscopy room),

postprocedure (up to 14 days), and late (any time after 14 days). For delayed events, the number of days after the procedure should be documented.
4. Events should be documented as: definitely attributable, probably, possibly, and not attributable.
5. Severity is graded by the degree of consequent disturbance to the patient and any changes in the plan of care. Adverse events should be followed until their conclusion to assess severity, and which should include the outcome of any new procedures required to treat them. Thus death after surgery for debridement of post-ERCP pancreatitis would be attributable to the ERCP. However, this should not apply to adverse events occurring after second procedures done solely because of the technical failure of the initial endoscopy (ie, without any adverse event prompting failure or abortion of the procedure).
6. Event tracking. Attempts should be made to contact patients at about 14 days after procedures to determine whether any adverse events have occurred, and whether they are attributable. Report generators should allow these data to be included as an addendum to the endoscopy report, including the statement that there were definitely no adverse events, when this had been confirmed by patient contact.
7. Reporting statistics. When reporting "complication rates," only definite and probably attributable events occurring within 14 days should be included. Rare adverse events that present after 14 days and are clearly attributable can be recorded as a separate category. Examples include a proven nosocomial infection, or stent migration causing a new clinical problem, not just failure of the original treatment goal.
8. Incidents are unplanned events that do not interfere with completion of the planned procedure or change the plan of care, that is, do not fulfill the stated criteria for adverse events. Examples include bleeding that stops spontaneously or with endoscopic therapy, and transient hypoxia that resolves with or without reversal agents, supplemental oxygen, or bagging. These incidents should be recorded for the purposes of quality improvement, and perhaps to see which incidents may predict later adverse events. Incidents may occur during the procedure or in the immediate recovery period (ie, while still under supervision).

Risk factors for adverse events

It is self-evident that adverse events are less likely to occur when both the endoscopist and the patient are well prepared for the specific procedure, and if performed with the support of a competent team in an appropriate environment. Issues relating to endoscopist and unit competence have been addressed earlier.

Understanding the risks inherent in specific contexts, and how to defuse them, was addressed recently by another working party of the ASGE. The goal was to examine the evidence for specific risks and to suggest a list of factors that might be included in endoscopy reporting/database systems. The conclusions of a very comprehensive review by Romagnuolo and colleagues were published in 2 parts, relating respectively to the risks for cardiopulmonary events[32] and the remainder, which relate mainly to individual procedure types.[33]

The factors increasing the risk of cardiopulmonary events are obvious, and include advanced age, established cardiac and pulmonary disability, other comorbidities, and obesity. These considerations and a few others are nicely wrapped up in the ASA score, which is a standard entry in most reporting systems. Risk is also affected by the setting for the procedure (eg, intensive care unit), its duration, and who administers the sedation/anesthesia.

There are many generic risk factors that apply to all types of endoscopy, including the type and complexity of any therapeutic activity, active infection, immunosuppression, and spontaneous or therapeutic coagulation deficits. ERCP carries other very specific risks, such as pancreatitis, the predictors for which have been widely researched and documented.[9,26,27]

Managing adverse events

There are several rather obvious but important management strategies when things "go wrong." The author believes that it is important to:

1. Recognize the problem quickly, and take appropriate diagnostic and therapeutic actions. Consult other specialists quickly as needed, especially surgeons when there is possibility of perforation (preferably one who knows that not all perforations need surgery).
2. Behave professionally, just as you would if things had gone well. Visit regularly, but not excessively. Explain carefully to the patient and family what has happened, referring to the consent process: "The x-ray shows a small perforation. You remember that we discussed that possibility beforehand. I'm sorry that it happened to you. This what we plan to do."
3. Show that you care. Saying "sorry" is simply to show sympathy, not to suggest that you did something wrong. Do not speculate that "I must have pushed too hard or cut too far." Keep in touch even if a patient is transferred to another service or hospital. Failure to do so may look like abandonment, and can make people angry and out for revenge. One way to show that you care is to give the patient your cell-phone number.
4. Ask whether there are other family members in the background (eg, nurses, paralegals) that would appreciate a phone call.

Benefits and Risks to ERCP Endoscopists

Endoscopists performing ERCP gain from their practice in several obvious ways, but they are also exposed to significant risks.

Physical harm

Radiation is an obvious hazard, although no definite damage has been described. It is wise to wear special spectacles, thyroid collars, and wrap-around aprons, and to monitor exposures. Endoscopists performing large numbers of complex ERCPs, and their assistants, should seek professional help from radiation safety officers to further minimize their exposure with customized barriers, such as lead-lined curtains and glass dividers on wheels. The chance of being infected by patients should be eliminated by standard shielding methods. Several surveys have shown significant musculoskeletal issues in endoscopists. Neck problems are more common in older endoscopists who practiced before videoendoscopy, caused by having to crouch over the eyepiece. Some ERCP practitioners have suffered from "cannulator's thumb" from working the elevator lever.

Medicolegal hazard

ERCP is the most dangerous procedure that endoscopists perform on a regular basis, and some bad outcomes are inevitable. Whether any of these lead to lawsuits is determined by how well endoscopists follow the advice outlined earlier.[34] By far the biggest issue is communication, or lack of it, at all stages of the process. Informed consent is not a piece of paper; it means that the patient fully understands the potential benefits, risks, limitations, and alternatives, and has developed sufficient trust in the people involved to accept the entire package on offer, including the chance of a poor outcome. This process can be assisted by brochures, videos, and interactive Web sites, and by nursing assistants, but must involve an unhurried face-to-face meeting with the endoscopist.

Endoscopists who practice within the accepted standard of care and who communicate well before and after procedures may still get sued, and lose some sleep, but not the suit.

SUMMARY

The clinical role of ERCP has changed substantially and progressively over its 4 decades of use, largely as a result of enormous strides in noninvasive imaging and considerable improvements in surgical outcomes. In the early days, 80% success in removing bile duct stones endoscopically, with a mortality of "only" 1%, seemed almost miraculous. Now we have to strive for much better outcomes, which demands more extensive training and enough ongoing experience to maintain and enhance expertise. The days of the occasional ERCPist should be over, but they are not. There is an unnecessary burden of severe complications and resulting lawsuits, which could be reduced substantially if the procedure was concentrated in fewer hands.[24] This is not to say that all ERCPs should be performed in tertiary referral centers, because basic biliary services at least must be available in the community, for convenience and because they may be needed urgently. Time will tell whether we can reach a situation whereby benefits are maximized and risks are minimized for all patients.

REFERENCES

1. Quality and outcomes assessment in gastrointestinal endoscopy. American Society for Gastrointestinal Endoscopy. Gastrointest Endosc 2000;52(6): 827–30.
2. Baron TH, Petersen BT, Mergener K, et al. Quality indicators for ERCP. Am J Gastroenterol 2006;101:892–7.
3. Cohen S, Bacon BR, Berlin JA, et al. NIH State of the Science Conference Statement; ERCP for diagnosis and therapy. Gastrointest Endosc 2002;56:803–9.
4. Cotton PB, Romagnuolo J, Faigel D, et al, The ERCP Quality Network; a pilot study of benchmarking practice and performance. American Journal of Medical Quality 2012, in press.
5. Aabakken L, Rembacken B, Lemoine O, et al. Minimum standard terminology for gastrointestinal endoscopy. Endoscopy 2009;41(8):727–8.
6. Cotton PB, Hawes RH, Barkun A, et al. Excellence in endoscopy: toward practical metrics. Gastrointest Endosc 2006;63:286–91.
7. Cotton PB. Income and outcome metrics for the objective evaluation of ERCP and alternative methods. Gastrointest Endosc 2002;56(6):S283–90.
8. Petersen BT. ERCP outcomes: defining the operators, experience and environments. Gastrointest Endosc 2002;55:953–8.
9. Freeman ML. Procedure-specific outcomes assessment for endoscopic retrograde cholangiopancreatography. Gastrointest Endosc Clin N Am 1999;9(4): 639–47, vii.
10. Schutz SM, Abbott RM. Grading ERCPs by degree of difficulty: a new concept to produce more meaningful outcomes data. Gastrointest Endosc 2000;51(5): 535–9.
11. Cotton PB, Eisen G, Romagnuolo J, et al. Grading the complexity of endoscopic procedures: results of an ASGE working party. Gastrointest Endosc 2011;75: 868–74.

12. Jowell PS, Baillie J, Branch MS, et al. Quantitative assessment of procedural competence. A prospective study of training in endoscopic retrograde cholangiopancreatography. Ann Intern Med 1996;125:983–9.
13. Available at: www.conjoint.org.au. Accessed October 3, 2011.
14. ASGE. Methods of granting hospital privileges to perform gastrointestinal endoscopy. Gastrointest Endosc 2002;55(7):780–3.
15. Cotton PB. How many times have you done this procedure, doctor? Am J Gastroenterol 2002;97:522–3.
16. Johanson JF, Cooper G, Eisen GM, et al. American Society of Gastrointestinal Endoscopy Outcomes Research Committee. Quality assessment of ERCP. Endoscopic retrograde cholangiopancreatography. Gastrointest Endosc 2002;56(2): 165–9.
17. Kapral C, Duller C, Wewalka F, et al. Case volume and outcome of endoscopic retrograde cholangiopancreatography: results of a nationwide Austrian benchmarking project. Endoscopy 2008;40:625–30.
18. Enochsson L, Swahn F, Amelo U, et al. Nationwide, population-based date from 11,074 ERCP procedures from the Swedish Registry for gallstone surgery and ERCP. Gastrointest Endosc 2010;72:1175–84.
19. Loperfido S, Angelini G, Benedetti G, et al. Major early complications from diagnostic and therapeutic ERCP: a prospective multicenter study. Gastrointest Endosc 1998;48:1–10.
20. Freeman ML, Nelson DB, Sherman S, et al. Complications of endoscopic biliary sphincterotomy. N Engl J Med 1996;335:909–18.
21. Rabenstein T, Schneider HT, Nicklas M, et al. Impact of skill and experience of the endoscopist on the outcome of endoscopic sphincterotomy techniques. Gastrointest Endosc 1999;50:628–36.
22. Available at: www.thejag.org.uk. Accessed October 3, 2011.
23. Cote GA, Keswani RN, Jackson T, et al. Individual and practice differences among physicians who perform ERCP at varying frequency: a national survey. Gastrointest Endosc 2011;74(1):65–73.
24. Cotton PB. Are low volume ERCPists a problem in USA? A plea to examine and improve ERCP practice—NOW. Gastrointest Endosc 2011;74:161–6.
25. Varadarajulu S, Kilgore ML, Wilcox CM, et al. Relationship among hospital ERCP volume, length of stay, and technical outcomes. Gastrointest Endosc 2006;64(3): 338–47.
26. Cotton PB, Garrow DA, Gallagher J, et al. Risk factors for complications after ERCP: a multivariate analysis of 11,497 procedures over 12 years. Gastrointest Endosc 2009;7:80–8.
27. Cotton PB. Risks, prevention and management. In: Cotton P, editor. Advanced digestive endoscopy: practice and safety. Oxford (England): Blackwell Publishing; 2008.
28. Fleischer DE, Van de Mierop F, Eisen GM, et al. A new system for defining endoscopic complications emphasizing the measure of importance. Gastrointest Endosc 1997;45:128–33.
29. Cotton PB. Outcomes of endoscopy procedures: struggling towards definitions. Gastrointest Endosc 1994;40:514–8.
30. Cotton PB, Lehman G, Vennes J, et al. Endoscopic sphincterotomy complications and their management: an attempt at consensus. Gastrointest Endosc 1991;37: 383–93.
31. Cotton PB, Eisen GM, Aabakken L, et al. A lexicon for endoscopic adverse events: report of an ASGE workshop. Gastrointest Endosc 2010;71:446–54.

32. Romagnuolo J, Cotton PB, Eisen G, et al. Identifying and reporting risk factors for adverse events in endoscopy. Part 1: cardiopulmonary events. Gastrointest Endosc 2011;73:579–85.
33. Romagnuolo J, Cotton PB, Eisen G, et al. Identifying and reporting risk factors for adverse events in endoscopy. Part II: non-cardiopulmonary events. Gastrointest Endosc 2000;73:586–97.
34. Cotton PB. Twenty more ERCP lawsuits: why? poor indications and communications. Gastrointest Endosc 2010;72(4):904.

Index

Note: Page numbers of article titles are in **boldface** type.

Gastrointest Endoscopy Clin N Am 22 (2012) 601–611
http://dx.doi.org/10.1016/S1052-5157(12)00080-3
1052-5157/12/$ – see front matter © 2012 Elsevier Inc. All rights reserved.

giendo.theclinics.com

Moving?

Make sure your subscription moves with you!

To notify us of your new address, find your **Clinics Account Number** (located on your mailing label above your name), and contact customer service at:

Email: journalscustomerservice-usa@elsevier.com

800-654-2452 (subscribers in the U.S. & Canada)
314-447-8871 (subscribers outside of the U.S. & Canada)

Fax number: 314-447-8029

Elsevier Health Sciences Division
Subscription Customer Service
3251 Riverport Lane
Maryland Heights, MO 63043

*To ensure uninterrupted delivery of your subscription, please notify us at least 4 weeks in advance of move.

Printed and bound by CPI Group (UK) Ltd, Croydon, CR0 4YY

03/10/2024

01040458-0004